Every Wall a Door

Every Wall a Door

Exploring Psychic Surgery and Healing

Anne Dooley

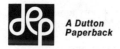 *A Dutton Paperback*

E. P. DUTTON & CO., INC., NEW YORK
1974

This paperback edition of

EVERY WALL A DOOR

First published 1974 by E. P. Dutton & Co., Inc.
All rights reserved. Printed in the U.S.A.
Copyright © 1973 by Anne Dooley

FIRST EDITION

10 9 8 7 6 5 4 3 2 1

Published simultaneously in Canada by
Clarke, Irwin & Company Limited, Toronto and Vancouver

ISBN 0-525-47380-7

Contents

Acknowledgments

I would like to express my thanks to Mr Maurice Barbanell, Editor of *Psychic News*, for his permission not only to make direct quotations from his newspaper but also to draw upon my own experience as a reporter in the years 1963–6.

I must also express particular thanks to authors (and/or their publishers) who have given me permission to quote extracts from their works: Geraldine Cummins, *Unseen Adventures* (Hutchinson); *Swan on a Black Sea* (Routledge & Kegan Paul); Granada Publishing and MacGibbon & Kee for permission to quote from Granada Guildhall lectures, 1965; Sir Alister Hardy, *The Living Stream* (Collins); Peter Hurkos, *Psychic* (Arthur Barker); Bernard Hutton, *Healing Hands* (W. H. Allen); Raynor Johnson, *The Light and the Gate* (Hodder & Stoughton); Julian Duguid, Editor of *Light*, for permission to quote Dr Oscar Parkes (May 23, 1935); Peter G. Sainsbury, Editor of the *London Hospital Gazette*, for a quotation from Vol. LXXI, No. 1, March 1968; Pedro McGregor, *The Moon and Two Mountains* (Souvenir Press); Jane Sherwood, *The Psychic Bridge* and *The Country Beyond* (Hutchinson); *The Fourfold Vision* (Neville Spearman); and S. M. Shirokogoroff, *Psychomental Complex of the Tungus* (Routledge & Kegan Paul).

1. Psi's Coming of Age in the West

On October 12, 1965, London's ancient Guildhall was packed to capacity for the century's strangest coming-of-age celebration: official recognition of the infant science of parapsychology or extra-sensory perception, variously and popularly referred to as psi, ESP, the supernormal or the supernatural.

Rarely in its long history has the City of London, backed by British Association scientists (headed on this occasion by Lord Brain as host of ceremonies), prepared a finer welcome for a transatlantic lecturer. He was Dr Joseph Banks Rhine, whose forty years' researches as head of the Parapsychology Laboratory at Duke University, North Carolina, U.S.A., have done so much to place telepathy squarely on the scientific map.

Psi is notoriously controversial and that evening proved rich in historic irony. Outwardly the stage was splendidly set; red carpets, striped awnings, cascading platform roses and a vociferously welcoming public whose pavement cheers turned to protest chants when the Guildhall's massive doors were eventually closed against a disappointed 200 overflow.

The address given that evening by seventy-year-old Dr Rhine opened the seventh annual series of Guildhall lectures jointly organized by the British Association and Granada Television "for the advancement of Science". His lecture was titled: "ESP—What Can We Make of It?"

Yet on that notable occasion I must confess I was both puzzled and disappointed by the famous researcher's unexpectedly tepid phrasing and occasional stumbling, almost embarrassed manner of delivery. My bewilderment increased the following morning when I found that *The Times*'s printed report differed rather radically in substance from my own shorthand transcript of the

9

delivered lecture. When I telephoned Granada's press spokesman to inquire about these mysterious discrepancies, I was told that Rhine had "modified" his original script. I was recommended to "follow my own notes".

My subsequent attempts to make direct contact with Dr Rhine before his departure for Paris and Prague proved fruitless. Further inquiries elicited from a sponsor that Rhine's original lecture had been considered "far too complicated". I was also told he had been "asked to use more day-to-day language".

The mystery was cleared up when I finally got hold of a proof copy of Rhine's original script, later published in booklet form at the end of the series.* The text not only explained the source of *The Times*'s own summary but also turned out to be substantially superior in style and content to the actual public lecture. The terminology was also well within the comprehension of any layman of average intelligence. So the question remains, *who* gave Rhine such unfortunate advice?

Both in his address and in his manuscript Rhine had dealt with the two main causes for the slowness of advance in psychic research. These related in part to orthodox caution, but primarily arose from the fact that psi was elusive and sporadic in its manifestations. The psychic sense, he told us, operated on such an unconscious level that even highly gifted subjects were frequently unaware as to whether they were scoring above or below chance rates in laboratory test runs. It was in the cogency of the revolutionary challenge presented by psychic phenomena that Rhine had departed most dramatically from his prepared script. In his script, which delineates the formidable obstacles which will stand in the way of the scientific control and practical application of psi ability, his conclusions are forthright.

Asking, "How conclusive is the case against a physical theory of psi?" he tells us bluntly that no valid evidence exists that definitely links a known physical energy to success in controlled psi tests.

He agrees that formidable problems stand in the way of psi application at present, but he remains undaunted.

Remarking that since all other sciences have always surpassed the wildest expectations of their founders, it is probable that in parapsychology, too, eventual conquests will surprise the world, Rhine makes the point that already, to some extent, psi *can* be

* The British Association/Granada Guildhall lectures 1965 (pub. Granada Television, distributed by MacGibbon & Kee).

controlled. He says, "We could have done little or no experimenting, if it could not."

Initially Rhine's method of clairvoyance testing was a fairly simple one, consisting of card-guessing tests using a special pack of twenty-five test cards consisting of five kinds of geometrical symbols as targets. The subject was informed of his scores immediately following a test run and was praised whenever he exceeded the chance average of five hits per run. Among the many student volunteers who tried their powers on these card-guessing tests sponsored by Rhine at the Duke Department of Psychology in the early 1930s was an exceptionally high scorer, a young man (H.P.) who was a Divinity School student. In the autumn of 1933 Rhine initiated a test he regarded as conclusive. The subject (H.P.) was put in a building 100 yards away from that of the experimenter. The two men worked with synchronized watches. Pratt* shuffled the cards just prior to the test and placed them, one at a time, face down on the table for one minute before removal. In this way a series of 12 runs through the cards was completed over a period of six days, the results being independently checked from duplicate records kept by both men. Rhine reports: "H.P. was found to have averaged 9.9 hits per run of 25 trials as against 5.0 to be expected from chance. The odds against chance producing so high a score are a hundred trillions to one."

Rhine later joined Pratt for a dual confirmation series of 6 runs through the cards when H.P. achieved an average of 9.7 hits per 25—the odds against chance here being a million to one.

In Rhine's view the tricky problem of control is "first and last a psychological one", which should yield eventually to sustained research. He pertinently reminds us that it must also be borne in mind that as yet not even a modest "crash programme" has been undertaken by any country or government.

Rhine, indeed, as a realist, places his greatest hopes for immediate progress in this field on the relentless competition between nations further to extend their mastery over physical nature.

In his concluding paragraphs he states with cautious optimism : "Even as I write these words there lies before me the announcement that a large American electronics company is engaging in a programme of parapsychological research, with the aim of

* J. G. Pratt, a distinguished psychic researcher and former collaborator with Rhine.

bringing ESP under practical control. One may infer with confidence that this indicates government interest and that some other government must be suspected of doing something similar. If that is not the case today, it will be so tomorrow.

"As it happens, then, behind the problem of advancing our knowledge of the human beings to whom psi belongs is a powerful practical interest with which we must reckon and for which we can even be thankful. And while this interest is due to nothing more than an overriding urge to get a man on the moon and especially to get one there first, presumably psi communication, if controllable, could be as useful in outer space as anywhere else man goes.

"At the very least, one must acknowledge the undaunted readiness of these technological professions for new and unconventional ideas. It is indeed conceivable that their purely practical interest may rocket basic research in parapsychology to an orbit of scientific atention it would not on its own attain within a century.

"This is not a note of cynicism, but simple recognition of the way things are. Let us recall that it was a very practical interest in the wine vats of France that started Pasteur's great revolution in medicine : it was not even a physician who led the way."

Already Rhine has proved to be a true prophet.

Rhine's intriguing reference linking American government interest in psi with the outer space race between the American and Russian governments to be the first to "get a man on the moon" probably linked with an earlier report presented in 1963 to the 14th International Astronautics Federation meeting in Paris. The speaker was Dr Eugene B. Konecci, chairman of its Bio-Astronautics Committee. His subject was telepathy, which he described as thought-transference over a distance, associated with the "non-demonstrable 'personal' psi-plasma field".

Referring to researches made by Soviet scientists, Konecci told his startled audience, "If the results of conducted experiments are half as good as some claim, then they may be the first to put a human thought into orbit or achieve mind-to-mind communication with humans on the moon."

He additionally confirmed that the telepathic race was also definitely very much *on* in America, and his report achieved headlines when he indicated that telepathically trained astronauts were not an unlikely possibility. He also revealed that the brilliant

American neurologist and psychic researcher, Dr Andrija Puharich, author of *Beyond Telepathy*, was likely to be given a chance to test out his exciting theory relating to evidence for what he termed a "Nuclear Psi Entity" in man in the form of "psi plasma" which he believes can exist independently of the physical body.

Puharich, incidentally, is also widening telepathic vistas in another most significant direction, for he appears to share the belief of Frederic W. H. Myers that telepathy is truly a cosmic law, capable of operating not only between the living but also between the living and the so-called dead. In his earlier, copiously documented book of psychic research, *The Sacred Mushroom*, which provides material as exciting as any first-class thriller, Puharich bluntly declared: "I do not doubt that discarnate intelligences exist, any more than I doubt that finite carnate intelligences exist. To me they are but opposite sides of the same coin. If we ever get complete understanding of one I believe we shall also understand the other."

Myers, of whom more anon, was probably the first man to point out that telepathy as a faculty must absolutely exist in the universe "if the universe contains any unembodied intelligences at all." After his death, unfortunately, there was a growing gulf between psychic researchers and those who believed in the hypothesis of survival, particularly Spiritualists. In effect, many reseachers complacently—but in my view, mistakenly—began to construe telepathy as a factor which *opposed* and largely cancelled out the possibility of post-death communication.

Research in consequence became increasingly bogged down in pompous and rather meaningless terminology increasingly directed towards the disparagement and refutation of mediumistic claims. As the psychic cold war deepened in fury in the opening decades of this century, the gulf continued to widen.

Rhine, however, has repudiated the suggestion that proof of telepathy necessarily rules out the hypothesis of survival. *Without* such proof, he says, it would not be possible to prove survival. Reminding us that the outstanding characteristic of ESP phenomena is "their failure to conform to the types of lawfulness expected of physical processes" he cogently argues: "In other words, here in the counter-hypothesis (to survival) itself is the kind of evidence that mankind has been seeking in the investigation of spirit communication—evidence of another order of causality but one that is, none the less, real for all its defiance of physical explanation."*

Certainly to an extraordinary degree Rhine's published thesis and the memorable Guildhall meeting, backed by British scientists, undoubtedly represented a great watershed in the century-old history of Western parapsychical research.

Although the *nature* of the energy behind psychic phenomena has remained so far uncharted by science, Rhine's brilliant summation of forty years' laboratory research revealed that within the span of a man's lifetime the emphasis had already switched from the former nineteenth-century research target of establishing the *factual existence* of psi's astonishing, apparently science-defying manifestations, to the new twentieth-century target of achieving *eventual control* of Man's increasingly demonstrable and mysterious sixth sense.

When Rhine addressed that large audience of scientists and researchers, less than seventy years had passed since the aforementioned Frederic Myers, a leading member of the brilliant team of Cambridge researchers who eventually founded London's Society for Psychical Research in 1882, had written its two-volume classic : *Human Personality and Its Survival of Bodily Death.*

Today, Myers' percipience of genius is being increasingly endorsed by outstanding scientists and researchers in ever widening fields. Only a few months after Rhine's memorable Guildhall lecture I was privileged to meet Sir Alister Hardy F.R.S., world-famed zoologist and marine biologist. It was the first interview he granted to a journalist after being elected President of Britain's Society for Psychical Research.†

Sir Alister told me : "Psychical research is as important for the future of mankind as the development of science itself has been over the past three hundred years. I made this point in my recent presidential address to the S.P.R. because I regard the solving of the mind-body relationship as man's most pressing need at the present time.

"What kind of future civilization we will have will depend on whether it is governed by a doctrine of materialism or not; that is why I regard our subject as of paramount importance."

He has enlarged upon this view in his widely acclaimed book, *The Living Stream,* which has provided a revolutionary "restate-

* "Science and the Spiritual Nature of Man" (*Fate,* U.S.A.), July, 1967.
† Published in *Psychic News* (June 11, 1966).

ment of the evolution theory and its relation to the spirit of man."
In it he makes a challenge to scientific orthodoxy:

> If only one per cent of the money spent upon the physical and
> biological sciences could be spent upon investigations of
> religious experiences and upon psychical research, it might not
> be long before a new age of faith dawned upon the world.

Like Myers and Rhine, Sir Alister regards telepathy as a factor
of crucial importance in biological evolution. In his chapter
"Biology and Telepathy" he tells how surprised his scientific
colleagues were when he had introduced the heretical subject of
telepathy into his Presidential Address to the Zoology Section of
the British Association at its 1949 meeting in Newcastle. Urging
them not to be ostriches in relation to riddling phenomena, he had
told them:

> There has appeared over the horizon something which many of
> us do not like to look at. If it is pointed out to us we say: "No,
> it can't be there, our doctrines say it is impossible". I refer to
> telepathy—the communication of one mind with another by
> means other than by the ordinary senses. I believe that no one
> who examines the evidence with an unbiased mind, can reject
> it.

Enlarging upon the "overwhelming evidence" bearing upon the
reality of telepathy, Sir Alister stresses the likelihood that it is of
widespread occurrence, though since it appears to operate in the
realm of the subconscious, only occasionally are a few unusual
individuals aware of it.

During the course of my own interview with Sir Alister at the
S.P.R.'s headquarters in London, I asked this seventy-year-old
genial giant of biology if he could enlarge upon his view that:
"The greatest obstacle to recognition of psychical research came
from biology itself."

He replied that this obstructing influence largely arose from a
widespread belief that acceptance of the Darwinian theory of

evolution "has shown that the whole process of life can be nothing more than a materialistic one".

Describing himself as being both a Darwinian and a Mendelian who also found thoroughly convincing the evidence for the reality of the D.N.A. chemical code governing heredity, he smilingly added: "I am, in fact, entirely orthodox in my evolutionary views, except that I do not believe that they yet tell us the *complete* truth about it all".

Full establishment of the reality of telepathy as a *scientific fact* would, he believed, do much to overthrow the still widely held view that mind was a mere appendage of the physical system, "reflecting events in the brain and nothing more".

He told me: "We really have no idea of the true nature of consciousness. I regard the pronouncement that the mind is simply reflecting what is taking place in the brain as a dogmatic statement for which we have no evidence. We must all have an open mind and go on examining the evidence."

Incidentally, in later correspondence with Sir Alister Hardy in January 1966, he wrote to me: "As you have gathered I really feel myself convinced that extra-sensory perception is not brought about by any physical radiation at present known to science, and I think it most likely it is something quite outside what we call the physical system."

Pascual Jordan, of Gottingen University, Nobel prizewinner and one of the world's leading atomic physicists, has endorsed this view.

Pascual Jordan was aware of the pioneer work in the early twenties carried out by the great Russian researcher and physiologist Professor V. M. Bechterev, who initiated telepathic research in his country and founded the Leningrad Institute for Brain Research.

How delighted he must have been when, in September 1962, the distinguished pupil of Bechterev, Prof. L. L. Vasiliev, Professor of Physiology in the University of Leningrad, published his scientific account of follow-up experiments which largely confirmed Pascual Jordan's own viewpoint.

Vasiliev's book, outlining the results of forty years' dedicated experimental investigations, is entitled: *Experiments in Mental Suggestion*. The subsequent authorized English translation meticulously carried out by two distinguished research-translators Anita Gregory and her husband C. C. L. Gregory, caused a furore among Western psychic researchers because Vasiliev described extensive experiments carried out in the thirties which had decisively refuted the earlier claim of F. Cassamalli, an Italian neurologist, that electromagnetic radiation was the medium of telepathic communication.

The investigation had been begun with the blessing of the Soviet government, for obviously had it been possible to establish that thought was transmitted by "brain wireless waves" then the scientific and philosophical basis of dialectical materialism would have been enormously enhanced. Vasiliev himself had commenced his initial $5\frac{1}{2}$ years' experiments with high hopes. He frankly confessed, "the results had surprised even those who were carrying out the experiments". He tells us: "Contrary to all expectation screening by metal did not cause any even faintly perceptible weakening of telepathic transmission. Even under conditions of double screening mental suggestion continued to act with the same degree of effectiveness as without screening. Is it necessary to emphasize that such a conclusion may be of tremendous theoretical importance?"

Fully cognizant of the anti-materialist implication of such a conclusion, Vasiliev and his co-workers undertook lengthy and arduous experiments in a vain endeavour to refute their own embarrassing inferences.

His translators tell us: "The investigations were at first officially encouraged by the Russian government: however, when it became clear in 1937–8 that such mental influence *did* occur, but was neither impeded by distance nor, apparently, mediated by electromagnetic radiation, and that no standard physical explanation was available, the work was shelved—probably suppressed and not referred to again in Soviet literature until 1959, after rumours had been spread concerning American military and naval interest in such matters."

By an ironic twist of circumstances, these French-circulated "rumours", although officially refuted in Washington, provided the competitive spur which enabled Vasiliev adroitly and successfully to bring pressure upon the Soviet authorities to take constructive action.

In *Experiments in Mental Suggestion,* Vasiliev states that at the end of 1959 and at the beginning of 1960, R. L. Kherumian, a member of the Paris Institut Métapsychique, had sent him two articles describing alleged sensational experiments in mental suggestion, which were believed to have been carried out in the summer of 1959 aboard the American submarine, *Nautilus*.

This experiment showed, and herein resides its principal value —that telepathic information can be transmitted without loss through a thickness of sea water and through the sealed metal covering of a submarine—that is, through substances which greatly interfere with radio communication. They completely absorb short and partly absorb medium waves, the latter being considerably attenuated, whereas the factor (still unknown to us) which transmits suggestion penetrates them without difficulty. These results were obtained by the Americans a quarter of a century after our above-mentioned ones of the "Thirties", and fully confirmed them. The only improvements of the American experiments over ours were that the telepathic influencing spanned longer distances and overcame greater physical obstacles, i.e. the great thickness of sea water together with the metallic covering of the submarine.

Amusingly, Vasiliev reveals that he himself was well aware that the French reports had been promptly denied by American government spokesmen. In the concluding pages of his book he inserted a footnote which covered the contingency, but at the same time cryptically indicated that he was not unduly impressed by U.S. attempts to play down their official interest in psi.

But the important thing was that Vasiliev had won his point with startled Soviet authorities and had established definitively the importance of his own earlier researches. Controversy continues, but psychical research in the Soviet Union has once more become public and authorized, despite its uncomfortable beckoning perspectives.

By the time of Vasiliev's death in early 1966, three of his books on parapsychology had already become best-sellers, translated into English, French and Bulgarian. Although his researches had been suppressed for over twenty years under Stalin's rule, a 400,000 edition of Vasiliev's psychic trilogy had sold out as soon as it appeared in Soviet bookshops.

Psi is indeed a very surprising subject developing in very surprising directions. Who could have foreseen, for example, even fifteen years earlier, that America and Russia would each be subsidizing telepathic research as a possible useful tool in the race to supremacy, not only in the depths of the world's oceans where their nuclear submarine fleets face unusual communication obstacles, but equally in outer space with its even more tempting power prizes and outsize hazards?

And as Rhine himself has written : *

In the last years the Western world has had to revise its opinion of science in the U.S.S.R. Another further achievement connected this time not with the conquest of the Cosmos, but rather with the nature of Man himself, will have to be credited to Soviet science. But if most astrophysicists foresaw that the first human being to be sent into space would be sent by Russia— no Western parapsychologist ever foresaw that it would be a Russian University that would be the first to establish a state-financed laboratory. However, this is exactly what has happened on the initiative of Prof. L. L. Vasiliev, as holder of the Chair of Physiology, and a corresponding member of the Academy of Medical Science. The subjects of study of this laboratory are called "bioelectronics", "brain communications" or, more freely translated, "mental radio". . . .

And, in its February, 1968 issue, *Sputnik*, a mass circulation Soviet magazine, widely circulated in foreign language editions, quoted Alexei Gubko, a scientist in the Ukrainian Institute of Psychology, as stating : "Most scientists are now inclined to believe that the brain radiates a special, hitherto unknown, type of energy which serves as the carrier of parapsychological information." Gubko also quoted R. L. Kherumian's view : "One day the development of parapsychology will direct our civilization on to a new road."

I myself was privileged, in September, 1964, to be given eyewitness accounts of Soviet and Czech scientists' work in parapsychology when I interviewed Dr J. G. Pratt, of Virginia University, U.S.A., a former collaborator with Dr J. B. Rhine of Duke

* Appendix 7, "Experiments in Mental Suggestion"—extract from editorial article in the Bulletin published by Dr Rhine's Parapsychology Laboratory at Duke University, U. S. A. No. 57, May 1961.

University, during attendance at the transatlantic convention held in Christ Church College, Oxford, and organized by America's Parapsychological Association.

In the previous year Dr Pratt had visited Prague where he met the brilliant Czech researcher, Dr Milan Ryzl, who had achieved the distinction of being the first man in any Communist country to have been nominated for the 1962 William McDougall Award for Distinguished Work in Parapsychology. This has been described as "psi's equivalent to the Nobel prize".

Commenting on his visit to Ryzl and the latter's view that with the help of hypnosis it was possible to train extra-sensory perception, even in persons who never had any previous such ability, Pratt, who told me of his visits and co-operation in experiments, said: "It *may* be that it heralds a new look in telepathy, but we don't really know yet. We have certainly known for a long time that the personality of the experimenter makes a great difference, in the same way that the sitter plays an important role in the end result."

Pratt's caution regarding such hopes that telepathy can be demonstrated as repeatable at will proved well-founded. Two hours after my interview with Pratt, Dr John Beloff, in the regretted absence of Dr Milan Ryzl, presented a paper to the Oxford conference entitled, "Hypnotic ESP Experiments in Prague". He reports that the performance of Ryzl's "star" subject, who had been trained to a degree whereby he could consistently achieve "beyond-chance" scores over a period of three years, had apparently recently shown a marked decline. The reasons for this, said Beloff, were not yet known.

Later at the conference, when I interviewed the well-known British researcher, Dr R. H. Thouless of Cambridge University, I asked *his* view about Russian and Czech attempts to seek practical and social applications of "controlled" telepathy in the field of long distance and hypnotic experiments.

He told me: "I certainly don't think they are barking up the wrong tree. In scientific research you have got to bark up *every* tree."

Some fifteen months afterwards I had a further opportunity to hear at first-hand from a British journalist colleague and friend, Theo Lang, sensational evidence that "Iron Curtain" researchers appeared to share the view of Dr Thouless.

Lang frankly admitted to me that when he had initially

undertaken his European investigations into psychic research developments on both sides of the "Iron Curtain" he had done so with considerable initial scepticism, but he confessed: "I have come back with a bend in my policeman's mind. I was very much impressed and surprised by the scientific calibre and standing of the men involved in these probing-the-unknown experiments."

My critically-minded colleague, who later published his findings in a series of articles published by a leading Sunday newspaper,* told me how, after visiting Dr Milan Ryzl in Prague, he had journeyed to the Eastern borders of Czechoslovakia to inspect a scientific machine so top secret that he was the first visitor from Western Europe—and the first journalist in the world—to be allowed to see it.

The sophisticated, fraud-proof research machine which Lang was permitted by scientists to see successfully tested in the Hradec Kralove Department of Physiology, had been designed by an investigating team, headed by Dr Ctibor Veseley, a lecturer in electro-physiology, to test the theory of telekinesis which claims that Man can control the movement of physical objects from a distance *by the power of thought alone*. The machine which Lang saw had taken three years to build.

Outwardly simple: a fold of paper-thin copper balanced on the point of a needle and revolving light as air, was housed or boxed-in with "sterile non-magnetic walls". The electric motor that turned the revolving needle was also magnetically screened so that it could have no effect on the circling fold of copper. When in motion the revolutions of the copper fold were counted photo-electrically and recorded.

Dr Veseley's interest, Lang told me, had first been aroused when in 1962 Robert Pavlita, a middle-aged technician, had arrived from a remote town, Horice in north-east Bohemia. Pavlita brought a crude self-built machine. He claimed he was able to influence its performance merely by mentally concentrating and *willing* it to change its movements.

In the presence of Lang and the Czech scientists sitting six feet away from the laboratory-built experimental machine, Robert Pavlita demonstrated the truth of his earlier claim.

Concentrating his gaze on the revolving copper he *willed* it to stop. In six tests out of ten it slowed or stopped completely.

Dr Veseley told the British journalist: "We are only beginning.

* *Sunday Mirror*, January, 1966.

Come back in another three years and we might show you more. But even then we might be only beginning."

Lang was also told of another similar Czech experiment in Bratislava where a famous Czech physicist, Dr Julius Krmessky, claimed to have moved light objects, floating on liquid, in a predetermined direction by mental concentration.

Certainly the cosmic-sized vistas opening out in the present decade of Man's intensifying *Mind* Revolution outpace even his breath-taking technological aspirations expressed in projected planetary probes.

The English Scene

2. Jane Sherwood

Paradoxically, although in the black months following my husband's death when I lived on alone at our cottage I was greatly tempted to plunge into an exploration of Spiritualism, an obscure feeling of shame prevented my doing so. On one occasion, arriving back in London from a weekend visit to my brother's home in Norfolk, I had even got to the point of looking up the address of the Belgrave Square headquarters of the Marylebone Spiritualist Association, now renamed the Spiritualist Association of Great Britain. But as I waited my turn in an exceptionally long Liverpool Street station queue for the necessary tube ticket, I suddenly changed my mind. In a crazy way I reasoned that if there did exist some other world in which, incredibly, Pat survived, then he'd be vastly engrossed in it and wouldn't approve of my fooling around instead of getting on with my own job of living—the job in hand. He couldn't bear whiners. To him it would have been the coward's way out.

The second attempt to dabble in dubious waters ended even more ludicrously. Towards the end of the Old Shop period when I was still working with an Essex group of weekly newspapers, the young editor who had replaced Pat kindly offered me a press ticket for a London Spiritualist healing rally at the Albert Hall. I accepted it gratefully, but when the day came and I was already half-way across London on my journey to the hall, I suddenly realized I'd inadvertently left the admission ticket in a weekend bag. Crestfallen, I once more decided: "So be it. I'll work out my own salvation as long as I can, like the seed under snow. Pat will find his own way of communicating if he's still around." And I think he did.

The dragging months passed. Thanks to the good-hearted

efforts of our neighbour and journalist colleague who had formerly lived next door to us in Essex, I had left the cottage in August 1958 and taken a proffered job as a reporter in Crawley, Sussex. During weekdays I worked hard. Leisure was always the dreaded enemy so I endeavoured to fill up the unwanted hours by getting down to a second play and a Prague-based novel. It was all unavailing. The neurosis which inevitably resulted from my futile attempts merely to turn my back on death as a blank wall, finally reflected itself in a disastrous block so far as creative writing was concerned. I could still carry out my daily job assignments. After all, run-of-the-mill journalism is merely a rather better-paid form of bricklaying, or any other craft. Outside of hack work, however, I was stranded high and dry.

In desperation I hit upon the idea of trying to write a book about Crawley itself, based on a series of ten neighbourhood profiles. The town had news value in those days. The ancient Sussex hamlet which had formerly been a half-way stop for coaches travelling from London to Brighton—a medieval inn still survives in the picturesque High Street—was fast burgeoning into one of Britain's liveliest post-war examples of New Town programming.

Fate soon showed its hand, for in the process of inquiring into Old Town organizations I ran plump into a local Spiritualist group whose members promptly invited me to report upon weekly healing sessions conducted in a member's home.

When I unenthusiastically presented myself on the appropriate evening my hostess decided that I myself could do with a "spot of healing", for her kindly questioning had soon elicited that I was in a depressed state, sleeping badly and suffering from frequent headaches. I found myself sitting on a kitchen chair while the proprietor of a dry cleaner's shop, a genial, middle-aged man said to have "the gift", made "healing passes" around my head and neck. I had no faith in his well-meant ministrations but I must admit they proved beneficial. For the first time in months I enjoyed two successive nights of sound sleep without the help of sleeping pills.

But the event which made that night an unexpected turning point in my life stemmed from what seemed at the time a mere whim. Waiting for the session to come to an end so that I could interview participants and patients I casually scanned the group's lending library. It consisted of a few score volumes about

Spiritualism and associated subjects. I was given permission to borrow one or two, and selected at random from titles which attracted.

Of the three books chosen, two were valueless. The third, however, had me hooked. It chanced to be Jane Sherwood's *The Country Beyond*. Written by a woman widowed in World War One, it told how, after years of unavailing effort, she believed she had finally succeeded in making contact with the world which lies beyond death.

She had undertaken her quest because: "First and most urgently I wanted conviction by way of clear knowledge or experience that the human personality survived death, and that the strongly felt presence of my husband was no feeble trick of self-deception."

She had begun by reading Spiritualist literature, attending seances and seeking out mediums. None had brought conviction.

"I was left," she wrote, "with a fine confused mass of claims and assumptions which were not easy to sort or reduce to probabilities. For some time judgment had to be suspended while this extraordinary material was collected. There was evident in this the growth of a structure of sober theory rising among a confusion of scaffolding which masked and travestied its lines. Credulity, fantastic dream matter, marvel-mongering, along with the type of mind most pathetically easy to dupe by these, had reared this inconsequential surround. . . .

"The fantastic element was at first my chief stumbling block. I heard much talk of Red Indian Guides, Child Guides, Egyptian and Chinese Guides, but seldom or never of English Guides. Almost analogous, I thought, to the musical world where an English name is no advertisement. . . .

"Spiritualist literature was bewildering. A substantial theory was evident, but a lush emotional atmosphere characterized most of these attempts to picture the life of the blessed in their various spheres. . . . Descriptions of towns had the same fairy tale quality of gorgeous pageantry surprisingly invaded by visitations from angelic beings of higher spheres. It seemed a perfervid hotch-potch of mystery and imagination gleaned from every variety of romantic and esoteric literature, past and present. . . . One wanted bread and was given, not a stone but a custard pie."

Finally Jane decided to go it alone. She embarked upon a dangerous and protracted experiment to try to resume contact with her dead husband by using a planchette. This object is a tiny platform of thin wood supported by two wheels and a pencil. The pencil point traces any movements caused when a user's fingertips rest lightly on the planchette when it is placed on a sheet of paper on which the letters of the alphabet have been written.

A medium had advised her to try this way of developing a possible latent ability to produce the psychic phenomenon known as "automatic" or "transmitted" writing. Automatists, as they are often called, are people who, while in a mentally passive state, can write without consciously directing the pen. Spiritualists believe that writings so obtained can in many cases be attributed to spirit direction. Psychologists and psychiatrists, on the other hand, tend to dismiss the phenomenon as, at best, mere subconscious thoughts and fancies. Dogmatism in either direction is dangerous, for both schools of thought leave largely unexplained the manifold inspirations of genius in many fields, not excluding mathematics, science and technology, of which more later.

Jane's own surprising experiences have been incorporated in a series of extraordinary books which provide more compulsive reading than works of fiction. One is the aforementioned *The Country Beyond*; another, her first book, is called *The Psychic Bridge*.

In the latter she describes her quest as, "A strange and fateful journey of exploration into queer byways of human experience. It proved to be a detour away from accepted paths, at times a difficult and dangerous one, but always one which in interest and adventure excelled the safe highway."

When, after two years of fruitless effort, her "poised pencil at last moved of itself into intelligible words" she tells us she became aware of a "quiet and powerful personality whose crabbed script was quite strange to me. I had made contact, but with a stranger."

When I read the book it was this stranger, "G. F. Scott", who primarily interested me because of the crisp pungency of his contributions in the described, seemingly impossible, life-after-death discussions and experiments between a living woman and three "dead" men, one of them her first husband, Andrew.

Scott, it appeared, had died in a road accident. In one of his spirit communications he told her : "On a certain hard road was strewn the wreckage of two machines—one a thing of metal tubes and cylinders, and one of chemicals in organic formation. But all the activities that had been associated with that smashed body of mine had vanished as far as an observer on earth was concerned, that is *I* had vanished. Well, here I am, well and active and that used up machine of my body must by now be well on its way to dust."

He also reported that when he came to after the crash he couldn't get his bearings. He had found to his surprise that though he seemed to be lying by a roadside, unattended, uncovered and unable to move, he felt neither pain nor cold. He expected to wake up from a nightmare and find himself in hospital.

"I slept and awoke several times before the suggestion that I was actually 'dead' occurred to me, and even then it was some time before I forced myself to entertain it. So certain had I been of the annihilation of the self that even this shadowy form of life was an astonishing reversal of theory. True, the cheerful earth had vanished with a completeness that staggered me in conjunction with the undoubted fact of my own very vital continuance. For I was more than merely alive in an earth sense. I was thrillingly, tensely alive, with all my being accentuated, keyed up and emotionally charged as never before. I tested and savoured this quivering being, cabined no longer in dull constraining flesh, but flowing from me as though I was the centre of a power-house of life. My body was actual, yet weight and solidity had gone, movement no longer lifted inertial mass but was the thing it moved."

I liked, too, the wry commonsense of Scott's comment: "Theorizing will become unnecessary when the majority of mankind become able to register our presence and feel our activities around them. When it becomes an actual experience to see us and feel us we shall have to be accepted as facts, even if we cannot be fitted into a theory. The trouble is that, lacking the experience, no theory, however plausible, is really convincing."

Jane Sherwood's fantastic book haunted my mind and when I was later invited by Theo Lang to collaborate in background research for his "investigation into mediumship" we decided it might be a good idea to try to track down Jane Sherwood. It didn't prove easy. Her wartime publisher confessed he had never set eyes on her. "I do not know if she is alive or dead," he told me. "There are some uncollected royalties."

And a London bookseller, who specialized in publishing and selling psychic and occult books, enhanced my deepening interest by remarking: "It is a strange thing about Jane Sherwood's books.

When they were first published they didn't attract much interest. They lay on the shelves for years. Now they are out of print I am inundated by demands I cannot fulfil from researchers and scientists. It's puzzling."

Finally her publisher agreed to forward a letter to her last known address. She had apparently moved meanwhile. Weeks passed. I had given up hope of receiving any response. Then I received a brief letter in handwriting of meticulous neatness. She invited me to meet her when she next visited London to attend a Quaker committee on which she served. We met on August 5, 1959.

Talking to this shy, white-haired, perceptive woman proved to be something of a journalist's ordeal. It was rather like trying to make friends with a wild bird. One jarring note and I knew she'd be gone beyond effective reach, even if conventional politeness prevailed.

She told me how, in the lonely freedom of a remote, lamp-lit cottage in Radnorshire, where she had sometimes been snowed-up for weeks at a time, she had penned her first manuscript, *The Psychic Bridge*.

"I have never told this to anyone before," she said, "but I was so inexperienced that I sent my original manuscript to a London publisher during the 1940–41 blitz. Weeks went by and receiving no reply from them I ventured to write. They replied that they had been glad to hear from me because a bomb had razed their offices to the ground, destroying all records and manuscripts. They asked me to send another copy. Of course I had none, so after I had recovered from the blow I had to sit down and painfully piece together my original notes and to write it all over again."

In the first two years of her experimenting she had set aside a daily period when she sat alone, hoping in vain for the "miracle of direct communication". When I asked her how she had found the courage to sustain the uncanny ordeal, she smiled, and replied: "If your purpose is sufficiently intense you keep on."

When a friend lent her a planchette she had regarded it as only "a silly toy". At first the results seemed mere gibberish, until, much later, she noticed with a slight interest that three initials G. F. S., which had no personal association for her, had become repetitive. Shortly before the overworked planchette collapsed the tracer pencil one evening moved right outside the circle of alphabet letters and the name G. F. Scott was written.

In *The Psychic Bridge* she records: "Curiously, hardly a doubt assailed me that an actual human entity was responsible for that signature. Experience has that indubitable seal of certainty about it quite impossible to convey, but completely efficacious in removing all doubts. I knew my search was over, and after the years of lonely experimenting, the shock of success halted me wordless. And there was more than this. I felt the impact of an emotion, a surprise and a joy that exceeded my own."

This self-taught woman has never received any scientific training yet her books have impressed scientists, including author-researcher, Dr Raynor Johnson, a British-born physicist and former Master of Queen's College, Melbourne University, who says Jane's theories range far beyond her own knowledge and conscious thinking.

In a preface which he later wrote for Jane's *The Fourfold Vision* (a study of consciousness, sleep and dreams) he tells us:

Some years ago I came across Mrs Jane Sherwood's book *The Country Beyond* and read it with a critical eye. No one who has read widely in the field of psychical research can be unaware of the problems and questions raised by automatic writing, but I must add that her book impressed me as a presentation of authentic communication. I regarded this book, and still do, as one of the best attempts to convey to us valid impressions of the conditions which we shall all have to meet some day when we have finished with our physical bodies. The same communicators, E. K. (a mature soul) "Scott" which is a pseudonym for another friend who desires to remain anonymous, and the writer's husband have collaborated further with Mrs Sherwood to throw some light on the manifold problems of consciousness, especially as they are presented by the phenomena of sleep and dreams. The general viewpoint can be simply stated, and it is this; that the human psyche is in the normal state a blend of four types of consciousness associated with the physical, etheric, astral and "spiritual" levels of the person. While the two former remain associated closely throughout life, the principal phenomena of sleep and dreams can be interpreted in terms of separation of the two latter from the body and from each other.

Too poor to buy books she needed, Jane had used libraries

extensively to win needed knowledge. "When I visit a library I seem to be impelled towards the book I need for study," she told me at our first meeting.

Theo Lang, a sceptic, wrote in subsequent articles : "Jane Sherwood is not an emotional or immature woman. There is obviously not a shred of superstition in her make-up. She is a calm and talented person. She is certainly completely sincere in her belief that she has established contact with her husband."

Referring to difficulties she had experienced in trying to publish later manuscripts relating to her two-worlds discussions, Jane Sherwood said : "I seem to fall between two stools. The religious people don't like my work and it seems I can't interest scientists either, although I am convinced that the mystery of what happens at the moment of so-called death *can* and will be explained scientifically, even if it takes another Einstein to achieve it."

She warns others who feel they, too, must seek direct experience in the psychic field : "Always retain your critical faculty. Even now, after all these years I am sometimes doubtful, though conviction does grow."

There is no easy path for any quester into mysteries of the psyche. For Jane the road, though hard and not without peril, has proved rewarding. She told me : "For years I, too, wanted to die. Now I have lost that feeling for I know there is work to do."

Adjourning to a London café we chatted about the identity of the lively, laughing communicator known under the name of "Scott". I confessed my exceptional interest in his personality. She laughed and suddenly asked : "Have you any idea who he might be?"

Normally I am about as psychic as a block of wood, but on this occasion, in the very act of preparing to shake my head in the negative, I felt as if an inner blinding ray of light had unexpectedly supplied an answer. With some embarrassed hesitance I found myself replying : "Perhaps I do. Is it T. E. Lawrence?"

Taken aback, and obviously regretting her indiscreet question to a journalist whom, after all, she had only met for the first time that afternoon, she replied, after a perceptible pause, "Yes."

Hastily reassuring her that I would not dream of betraying a personal confidence, I said : "It's so odd that it should be Lawrence of Arabia, because it so happens there is a link with my husband."

After I had told her my strange story she leaned back in her chair and laughed rather ruefully. "I am not sure I like it," she said. "I think we are being used."

Some of the events I recalled extended over thirty years. Born in an ugly, hard-hit Yorkshire mining village, son of an Irish miner, Pat had been sent down the pit at the early age of 13. Shut away from the sun, and hating his claustrophobic hardships, he had tried to continue his scant education by reading a page of the dictionary daily during his "snap" breaks. He eventually ran away and joined the army. By some strange chance he enlisted in the same Dorset-based battalion in which "Lawrence of Arabia" was then serving as "Private Shaw".

Sensing the teenager's hunger for knowledge, Lawrence had been kind to him and other young recruits. For many years my husband cherished the "book list" drawn up for him by "T. E.", and a small pen-and-ink drawing given to him by Lawrence after Pat had admired it.

It was also in Lawrence's nearby cottage that the young ex-miner ate his first olive, listened to classical records played on the hand-built gramophone his host had designed, and saw the Augustus John murals charcoaled on hessian drapes, providing one of the few art luxuries in T. E.'s hermit retreat.

After a short period their paths sharply diverged. They never met again, though the memory of T. E.'s spontaneous kindness endured in the memory of the younger man.

What impressed me so deeply when I pondered Jane's revelation was the fact that since at that time I had no Spiritualist acquaintances, no alternative avenue had been left open for any link to be made between the worlds separating Pat and myself.

Strangely, too, Jane had been drawn into her own direct investigations by a similar, seemingly planned "link". In *The Psychic Bridge* she tells how, after a long interval, she had renewed correspondence with a friend of her younger days and eventually spent part of a summer holiday with her. During the holiday the friend had, with some embarrassment, told Jane:

"I have for a long while been hesitating before delivering to you a message which came some months ago at a seance to which I had escorted mother. I was not supposed to be taking part and sat out of the circle. The medium was in trance and at the end of the sitting she insisted there was a message for me from a soldier. I protested I had no friends in the forces. She urged that the message was important, she added that it was not for me personally but for a friend I should soon be meeting. As you know, you and I had neither met nor written for two years so you were not in my mind."

Jane was both impressed and puzzled. The given message included details which, she tells us, "showed a clear knowledge of all that had befallen me since Andrew's death. It was as though, fumbling blindfold in the fog, a hand had suddenly clasped mine to assure me I was not searching alone."

She also wondered how he could have known so surely that the friendship would be renewed. "I checked on that—the advance had come, not from her, but from me. I had suddenly found myself thinking of her, had guiltily realized my neglect to write and had been impelled to renew the correspondence. . . . Was all this coincidence, or a deliberate impressing of my mind by Andrew?"

Jane, like myself, had reviewed her own circle of friends and realized that the one who had been given the unexpected message was literally the only one who maintained contact with Spiritualist circles, "absolutely the only channel through which any such message could have reached me."

When Jane finally made her own direct contact with her dead husband he had described the difficulties he had experienced in achieving longed for contact with the earth from *his* world.

"I had hoped to reach you directly but soon found I couldn't make you understand me. . . . For years I gave it up because there was great difficulty in finding you. Then I made another attempt. . . . There was a chance that in your own district some Spiritualist gatherings might be held which would provide a means of getting a message through to you. I knew some people here who were acting as Guides and made enquiries among them. They knew the names of the places and of some of the people with whom they came in contact.

"I can give you the name of the medium who took my message. She was a Mrs H. and her Guide knew some of the people she visited. They included the familiar surname of your friend, someone living in your district, so I took a chance on that. . . . *It's as much an organized affair* on our side as it is for you. How else do you think any connection could possibly be made?"

Not surprisingly perhaps but very happily for me, Jane and I became friends. On a 1959 visit by Jane to my Crawley home I was permitted to read T. E.'s posthumous journal, transmitted through her pen and hand. The experience deepened my now keen interest in psychic matters and strengthened my own determination to continue the quest for Survival proof. I did not have to wait very long.

At a trance sitting with Douglas Johnson I asked the "communicator", said to be my husband, if he had met T. E. Back came the answer: "Yes, but he is in a different part to me—a step up the ladder."

In March, 1960, at a second trance sitting with another well-known British medium, John Lovette, I was told: "Your husband is laughing about a 'T. E.' He's saying, 'He is a mystery man'." Later mention was made about T. E. and Pat "working in the same Group".

From time to time, at infrequent sittings with these two brilliant mediums I continued to be given brief greetings and encouragement from T. E., but, like Jane Sherwood in her early psychic questing, I was never quite convinced.

In 1963, after a period of carrying out part-time freelancing and book reviewing for Britain's Spiritualist news-weekly, *Psychic News*, I accepted a full-time job on the paper. Events again quickened in the links so mysteriously and inexorably being forged between a very contrasting foursome comprising T. E., Jane Sherwood, my husband and myself.

Six weeks after our first meeting Jane herself had taken steps to find out a little more about the chain of circumstances which had led to our own meeting. In September 1959 she wrote to me:

"I had a communication from 'Scott' yesterday and I told him of the connection with your husband. He said: 'I remember him. It's certainly a curious coincidence. *I* don't arrange these things but I have learned enough to discount coincidence—there is a plan. It's just as likely that the encounter was engineered by Pat but I'll try to find him and let you know.'"

There the matter rested. It seemed as if once again the curtain so tantalizingly momentarily lifted between the two worlds of the living and the "living-dead" had inexorably come down. It proved not to be so for another glimpse was proffered in a very unexpected manner.

On January 29, 1964 I chanced to consult a London publisher, Neville Armstrong, about some research I had just undertaken on a fringe subject related to parapsychology. In conversation I happened to remark upon his own seeming interest in the subject, judging from one or two psychic "titles" I had spotted in his publisher's list. He briskly assured me that he only published "very exceptional books on the subject".

On impulse I suggested he should read Jane Sherwood's manuscript relating to Lawrence of Arabia's posthumous communications. Two years earlier I had been instrumental in helping to get these serialized in *Psychic News* but they still awaited publication in book form. He agreed and I sent him the manuscript. Three days later he excitedly telephoned me : "I read it at one go," he said. "I've decided to publish it."

His decision led to a rather astonishing postscript some weeks later when I was invited to attend a memorable Good Friday voice seance in John Lovette's flat. It was my first experience of direct voice, that now rare psychic phenomenon in Britain.

Eleven sitters closely encircled the entranced man in the cramped confines of a medium-sized room during a fantastic three hours' seance when spirit voices—each in their own fashion —appeared successively to proclaim, "We live, we live." They spoke through a luminously-painted trumpet which repeatedly rose unsupported from the ground, slowly travelling at waist height round the circle of sitters until "they" had found the right recipient for particular messages. It was uncannily as if dead matter had become momentarily and incredibly imbued with gravity-defying intelligence and purpose.

The gramophone-accompanied proceedings had been prefaced by an explanation from the entranced medium's "spirit" master-of-ceremonies. For the benefit of newcomers like myself he explained that it was a mistake to believe that in a direct voice seance you heard "the actual voice of the communicator". He described the need to build a "voice box" with ectoplasm* drawn from the bodies of the medium and the sitters.

The brief explanation was followed by what I can only describe as an astonishing display of psychic pyrotechnics. By the light of a

* Ectoplasm (from the Greek *ektos* and *plasma*): exteriorized substance described by Swedenborg as "a kind of vapour steaming from the pores of my body".

red paper-covered torch held in the medium's hands, sitters witnessed a foaming "river" of ectoplasm extending from his mouth to the floor. Within seconds it was variously shown, at first diaphanously covering his body with the torch shining through it, then a moment later it extended across a neighbouring divan. The final "flash" showed the complete disappearance of the ectoplasm, within a split second of it having been piled on the floor in front of the medium. The medium himself, wedged between gramophone and divan, could not have made any untoward movement out of his chair without being spotted by one or more of the sitters who included three veteran journalists. One of them, seated next to me, was also a well-known author and sceptic, yet I observed later in the proceedings that he was obviously moved when a travelling trumpet, after "caressing" him in outline, suspended itself unsupported in mid-air before him. Through it a voice joyously proclaimed delight at "speaking for the first time to my son". He also unexpectedly received a message from a man who had committed suicide—Frank Tilsley, a former playwright and broadcaster. Tilsley reminded him of their last meeting. The journalist told me later that he and Tilsley had participated in a broadcast programme only three days before the tragic event. He confessed he had found the seance "a remarkable and moving experience".

My own turn to be startled came much later in the seance after I had witnessed a fascinating psychic ballet during which the flying trumpet (actually a cone-shaped megaphone) travelling at amazing speed, performed complex, ceiling-scraping arabesques, accompanied by a similarly airborne bell which ended its "dance" on the head of a middle-aged man seated to the medium's left. Wavering golden globular and zig-zagging lights had also circled above our heads, interspersed by chill perfumed "breezes" and a "baptismal" sprinkling of water at one point.

Efficiently completing the rapid demolition of a cynicism I had long entertained about the identity of the communicator who called himself "T. E.", the trumpet, resting mid-air in front of me, had announced : "This is T. E." To my startled, inane reply, "Oh, I've often wondered if you were *real*," the voice-from-the-dead mockingly countered : "Really ! And I don't mean that as a pun."

T. E. then proceeded to congratulate me on "the work you are doing," adding for good measure, "I've come to cement the link."

I can only tell you that none of the eleven sitters present, or the medium, could have known of the "work" to which the unseen communicator referred, for only a few days before that Lovette seance the publisher had telephoned to tell me : "The contract for Jane Sherwood's T. E. communications has now been signed."

3. The Strange Ones

If anyone had told me that in middle age I should one day find myself taking a 90-mile round trip in the forlorn hope of keeping a date with the dead I would have scoffed at a grim joke in dubious taste. Yet, on a sunny morning in 1959, this is precisely what I found myself incredibly doing when a freelance research assignment led me to the Brighton home of Douglas Johnson. This talented professional medium later won headlines in the national press following his first appearances on television in two widely discussed B.B.C. programmes, in the winter of 1960.

When I later wrote about that memorable encounter I told how I had found myself experiencing a very unprofessional feeling of trepidation as I neared my destination, a ground floor flat in a pleasantly quiet Edwardian terrace high above the sea. What was I going to find behind that gaily painted door? Anticipated bleak disappointment, or the dawn of a fabulous hope? One thing was certain: Mr Johnson and I were strangers to each other. My "sitting" with him had been booked days earlier by telephone; and, apart from my name and sex, he could know nothing of myself or my circumstances.

The relaxed, welcoming smile of the slender, keen-faced, dark-eyed man who ushered me into a comfortable sitting room furnished in unostentatious good taste soon put me at ease. When I rather diffidently asked permission to take notes during the sitting he pleasantly consented: "By all means. I only wish more sitters would do so." Many mediums find it is helpful in establishing initial contact, to hold some article belonging to the sitter. In this instance I handed to Mr Johnson the wristwatch I was wearing.

I am not likely to forget the next 45 minutes. As my pen raced over the paper to keep pace with the soft-toned, gentle voice, which soon gained speed and sureness, my whole consciousness became an astonished concentration upon what that voice was impossibly relating.

At one time or another in our lives most of us have engaged with our friends in semi-playful attempts to mind-read, even if we have only participated in that primitive form of group-tele-pathy, "Guess the object." It is a form of fun which usually soon palls from sheer frustration. But, as I now faced this stranger, who sat in a withdrawn stillness, it was as if an outer skin of my brain had been stripped away, enabling him to read fact after fact correctly, building a vivid picture of a shattered way of life, the manner of death of my husband, and his strongly individual character. Of 26 directly personal facts enumerated, facts which included the actual age difference between myself and my husband, his three-letter nickname, and a private joke about fishing, only one was incorrect—the actual date of his death.

Remarkably, too, one comment about which I demurred during the sitting later proved to be correct. The medium told me : "He's saying something about a Chinese drawing of a horse—is there some change in it? Have a look!" At the time of the sitting I was positive that the drawing remained untouched in a roll container placed by my husband in a bureau drawer about a year before his death. When I returned home and discovered that the "horse" was not among the three drawings originally placed in the roll, my first thought was that I had gifted it, in memory of my husband, to my brother who had admired it and who was one of the few people to have seen it. Inquiry proved this to be wrong; and to this day, despite probings of my admittedly bad memory, I still do not know what did happen to that cherished charcoal drawing.

It is difficult, also, not to be shaken, and quite impossible not to be deeply moved, when a stranger, in the course of an apparently fantastic trio conversation between himself, his "con-trol" and a dead man, suddenly relays to you phrases, comments, adjurations and endearments couched in precisely the vivid, characteristic expressions which would have been used in life.

At the end of the sitting, when I was recovering my temporarily lost composure by smoking a proffered, and much needed cigarette, I told Mr Johnson that I was a journalist carrying out a research assignment. I asked him if I might question him about aspects which puzzled me, and continue to puzzle me as I pen these lines.

"We are often told," I said, "that mediumship is largely telepathy or mind reading." He smiled and said mildly: "Well if so, can you explain to me how it is that during psychic research experiments—proxy sittings, for example, when I am handed a packaged article belonging to some person unknown to me, it is still possible for me to give information which is later verified as correct? And if it *is* only telepathy, can you also tell me why it is that we don't describe the living as often, or more often, than we describe the dead?"

Inwardly I commented to myself, touché, for I recalled that when I had earlier asked a well-known palmist if he could tell me the difference between fortune-telling and mediumship, he had unhesitatingly replied: "Ah, *we* don't see the dead. Our *gift* is clairvoyance and precognition."

Pursuing my questioning of Mr Johnson, I asked him: "Why is it that with some sitters you get what might be termed good results, while with others I am told you return your fee because you can get nothing?"

"Yes," he answered, "that's quite true. Some sitters I can do nothing with and I tell them so frankly. I find that it is the very 'cold' sitters who nearly always get poor results. I think that is why many so-called experimenters confess to disappointment. All I ask of any sitter is that they should keep an open mind and have a fair attitude. Some researchers, however, perhaps unconsciously, confuse a so-called scientific attitude with a hidden bias in favour of a so-called materialist philosophy. In consequence they are prejudiced and on occasion unduly suspicious." He added: "It is not sufficiently realized that the sitter himself plays an important role in the success or otherwise of a sitting. Fundamentally, much depends on the individual having somebody on the other side of life whom they love and who is interested in them. In life, if somebody close to you—say a mother, husband, wife or brother—goes to a distant country, then naturally you maintain contact by letter or telephone; but where the link or relationship is not strong the contact is not maintained. It is just the same with someone who has died. If there hasn't been, and does not exist, a strong affectionate link, why should these so-called 'dead' come through? They have their own lives to lead."

"People sometimes confuse fortune-telling and mediumship. Is there a close connection?" I asked.

"It is an interesting question," he said. "I, myself, believe that the psychic sense can operate on different levels. There is the level on which psychics who give material advice—fortune-tellers if you like—can operate. On this level you can get clairvoyance and precognition. By holding your watch, for example, I contact conditions and circumstances of importance in your life. I may even get precognition of future circumstances.

"Then there is the higher level when one feels in some way entirely different. One gets a feeling of peace and closeness to some different force and this, I believe, arises from the influence of one's helpers and advisers on the other side, and the resulting impact that comes, until you quite definitely begin to see things from a different angle. If I might so express it, instead of working on parallel lines, as in psychometry, I feel I am working perpendicularly, or, if you like, upwards. I believe it hits a different psychic sense, or at least a different level. You then become conscious of a sense of exhilaration. When there is a strong bond between a sitter and someone who has passed to the other side of life, and you are able to establish a good contact, you get almost a feeling of excitement and happiness. Most true psychics in such cases would willingly give sittings for nothing."

Time was speeding, so I put my final question. "We hear much about dishonest mediums and the dangers of self-delusion. Would you care to comment?"

"It is true," he told me, "there *are* fraudulent mediums, and every honest psychic welcomes their exposure. It is despicable to trade upon human sorrow and grief. This said, I do not believe that in general you will find a higher percentage of frauds in my profession than you would, say, among solicitors. A much greater difficulty for us is that it is sometimes far from easy to sort out where actuality ends, and imagination takes over. If you are a good psychic you are successful with many sitters, but it is when you begin to think you are infallible that the rot sets in. The medium must possess integrity and inner balance. It is also necessary to have a highly developed natural gift. You either have a gift to develop, or you haven't, just as you might have a gift in any other field—for mathematics or engineering.

"If you have a natural gift, with progress you gain confidence. At the beginning you sometimes hesitate over what you are getting because the message may seem to you absurd, or unusual and therefore you think it is wrong. But often it is the most seemingly ridiculous things which are the most evidential and striking. I was taught a lesson once. I had a sitter, a very nice woman in deep sorrow over the death of her husband. After the sitting, which she thought was a good one, she told me her husband had been interested in psychic things for many years. They had arranged a code which they thought would be easy to transmit. She said sadly that she had never received it. I replied: 'It is very strange, but these things do happen. What sort of code was it?'

" 'It was a pictorial code,' she said.

" 'Well,' I told her, 'the only picture I got seemed so silly I didn't pass it on. I saw your husband with a bowler hat sitting astride an elephant.'

"With a radiant smile she exclaimed: 'Oh, that's it.' I told her that probably other mediums she had visited might also have got the picture, but, like myself, had hesitated to describe it. I myself had happened to visit a circus the night before and thought it was only a jumble in my mind."

I came out again into the sunshine, and as I walked downhill to the mirror-bright sea I was a very thoughtful woman indeed. I still dared not be too confident that a phoenix had been born from the ashes of my despair, but at least I was certain that my journey behind the gaily-painted door had not yielded the chagrin of disappointment. Indeed, as I idly watched the soaring flight of a seagull above the summer sea I suddenly realized with a poignant shock that I was temporarily experiencing an almost forgotten sensation—happiness. It was as if my "date" with the dead had yielded me a momentarily radiant vision of a chink of light gleaming from beyond a hitherto obdurately closed door.

In subsequent years, as my personal and professional interest in psychic research steadily deepened, I was indeed fortunate in meeting many of Britain's best-known mediums, some of whom I count myself privileged to regard as friends. To all of them— sometimes in very unlikely circumstances when operation of the mediumistic gift would normally have been deemed impossible—I am indebted for a slowly accumulating and eventual astonishing abundance of evidential "communications" which finally toppled the last of my strongly entrenched doubts. Personal conviction, of course, is only important to the individual concerned. I have stated it here, not only as a necessary confession—if confession it be—of an unanticipated viewpoint tardily attained, but also to express my gratitude to those who made it possible. More important to readers of this chapter is that in the process of becoming convinced that we do survive physical death, I slowly gained an insight into some of the still little understood processes and life patterns which underlie the mysterious psi faculty when it is expressed in professional mediumship. This insight I owe entirely to the unusual opportunities richly afforded to any assiduous and sincere journalist-researcher. For this reason the material I present in these pages has value because it is not based upon my own conjectures but represents the experiences of outstanding mediums as they generously described them to me not only in formal interviews but also in friendly chats over the years.

Perhaps the most significant pattern to emerge—a pattern which confirms Douglas Johnson's view that mediumship is a specific, and frequently an inherited, talent—is the frequency of its manifestations in the early childhood of gifted sensitives.

Internationally famed veteran London medium Mrs Bertha Harris, for example, told me she could never remember a time in childhood when she had not been aware of what she terms "the little people". Indeed she took them so much for granted as being part of the everyday earthly scene that it was not until two terrible family tragedies occurred within months of each other that she suddenly realized that she had simultaneously been living in touch with two worlds, not one.

The knowledge first hit Bertha like a shock wave when, after only an hour's illness, her younger brother died in her arms. "When I saw his spirit body build up and heard him say, 'Isn't it strange, I am out of my body?' I suddenly realized that all the 'little people' I had been seeing must also have passed over." A few months later the same grief-fraught illumination was repeated when she watched her father die following an accident. "I saw his spirit leave his body and come and stand by me. Then I heard him say: 'Well, it's all over. I am all right'."

And she was still only a shy, leggy, 16-year-old when, on the platform of one of Manchester's biggest halls, she startled a 2,000-strong Good Friday audience by describing a tragedy she alone could perceive. She said a "spirit" communicator, a man who had formerly worked in Belle View Zoo, was "very upset because he now sees a little girl called Poppy going into a lion's cage with a skipping rope. What she is going to do is going to cost her father his life. He can see the lion coming forward. The father is trying to save his daughter but is hampered by a wooden leg."

No one claimed any knowledge of "Poppy" or her father. The

message appeared to be the one failure in an otherwise brilliant city debut. Next day, however, the morning papers confirmed the accuracy of her clairvoyance. The fatal accident had happened in a small touring circus which had set up its tent on waste ground just behind Manchester's famous zoo. Only ten minutes after the young schoolgirl had so dramatically talked about the spirit-witnessed accident, the mauled man had been rushed to hospital where he died of his injuries.

Another talented childhood visioner of the Unseen was Mrs Gladys Osborne Leonard who first achieved international fame as the medium used by Sir Oliver Lodge, scientist and psychic researcher. His weekly sittings with her commenced in 1915 after the death of his soldier son Raymond.

In her autobiography, *My Life in Two Worlds*, Mrs Leonard has vividly described her childhood psychic experiences. She wrote that :

Frequently, in whatever direction I happened to be looking, the physical view of the wall, door, ceiling or whatever it was, would disappear, and in its place would gradually come valleys, gentle slopes, lovely trees and banks covered with flowers of every shape and hue. The scene seemed to extend for many miles and I was conscious that I could see for many miles, much farther than was possible with the ordinary physical scenery around me.

And this modest, courageous woman who regarded herself merely as a "human telephone connecting you with another world" also assures us :

I myself have not found that the development of psychic awareness detracts in any way from other so-called normal studies. I am a more successful gardener than I used to be, I am a much better cook; in many ordinary but useful directions I know I have improved; my health and nerves are under better control and therefore they are more to be relied upon than they ever were before I developed what many people think of as an abnormal or extraordinary power.

Another medium with a powerful inborn psychic sense is my friend, Stanley Poulton. This pocket-sized dynamo with a sparkling zest for life, laughter and psychic crusading early became a star medium and the despair of reporters, for only a tape-recorder can keep pace with his evidential verbal flow when he is on a platform.

Like Gladys Leonard he, too, in childhood became haunted by the beauty of an unearthly landscape frequently glimpsed between the ages of five and eight. He told me that his recurrent vision, almost a daily occurrence in that three-year period, took the form of a large garden. "Although I would continue to remain conscious of my own everyday surroundings, it was as if a veil lifted. Suddenly I was also looking into another world where familiar colours glowed in greater depth than we know here. In front of a cottage in that garden, I always saw my silent friend, an elderly man of waxy appearance who used to come and stand by my bed at night when my elder sister read to me. Always a strange feeling of inner happiness accompanied the vision. When I stopped seeing it, it was like losing an old friend."

Stanley never told anyone of his secret until one day when—in his Other World garden—he suddenly saw an uncle coming towards him through the garden. "I ran inside and told my mother of our visitor. He didn't arrive and I was scolded for telling lies." But the uncle the boy had "seen" died suddenly six days later. Coincidence? Or previsioning? There was an equally intriguing sequel. Stanley told me that years later, after he had already become a well-established professional medium, he received another unexpected visit from his "dead" uncle. Tired at the end of a busy day Stanley had flopped into an armchair in his charming London home. "Suddenly the door opened and my uncle popped his head round it as he used to do when we were children. He looked so happy I got the strange feeling he had come to take my aunt 'home' with him. I couldn't shake off the premonition. I went to my parents' home and asked my mother if she had received any news from my aunt. My mother, a little surprised, told me she was quite well. A fortnight later, however, we received news of my aunt's passing."

Mrs Ena Twigg is another very talented medium who is so used to seeing "ghosts" in her eventful life that she is constantly being freshly surprised that other less gifted mortals like myself cannot see them too. She not only *sees* spirit forms of the living-dead but also hears them speak to her, as I can personally testify. On one notable occasion when she had telephoned me on a mundane matter she suddenly broke off, paused, then excitedly exclaimed: "Your husband is here. He's so clear, can't *you* hear him too? He wants me to tell you. . . ." Then followed an amusingly characteristic evidential message, topped off with a puzzling prediction and warning which, at the time, did not make sense to me. He foretold that I would very soon receive an unexpected job offer which I should turn down because I shouldn't made a break with present activities. Sure enough, three weeks later, out of the blue I received a job offer which was so attractive that had I not been earlier warned not to "make a break" I should undoubtedly have accepted it. Eighteen months later I understood the reason for my husband's Other World admonition, for had I not heeded his advice I would have missed out on one of the biggest adventures of my adult life, the out-of-the-blue meeting with Lourival de Freitas and subsequent journeyings which led to Brazil and this book.

When lecturing or demonstrating in public Ena, a petite, elegantly groomed woman, expresses a sparkling vitality which makes it seem incredible that she has survived more than one nine-round battle against death. Indeed, it was as a result of one of these grim encounters that she pledged to devote the rest of her life to helping the bereaved and sick through her mediumship. Following an emergency operation for appendicitis in the Mediterranean area she had reached England still gravely ill. Down to six stones in weight, and victim of successive heart attacks, the medical prognosis was not hopeful. Then came the "miracle" which proved to be a decisive turning-point in her life. One night she saw her bedroom door open and three spirit forms—an old man, a young man and a woman—approached her bed. The old man told her: "We have come to help you. Tell me all the illnesses you have ever had." After she had done so she felt as if an injection was administered in her arm and knew no more. Next morning when Ena told her husband of the strange happening he thought she was dying. "After this first visit they came regularly," she told me, "and I began to feel more cheerful. I ate more, started to meet people and began to get about. Then after six months they told me: 'Our job is done.' I asked how I could repay them. I was told, 'By giving to others what you have received'."

Questioned at a London meeting about the techniques of

mediumship, she humorously described herself as "a bit of a split personality. Sometimes in trance I feel I am 'out there' collecting a lot of information." Asked how she switched on, she replied: "Before a sitting I try to forget myself. You must not allow personal feelings to intrude. You must be disciplined. I always 'listen in' on my left-hand side. When I hear something there, I know it is going to flow beautifully." She also confirmed that when conditions at a sitting were favourable it was possible to experience "such an attunement between the unseen, the medium and the sitter that the feeling of two worlds vanishes. It is just like people laughing and talking together in the same room." A fascinating riddle of her mediumship is that when she foresees future scenes or events they invariably appear to her in colour. Of public clairvoyance she has stated: "I can remember times when I've stood absolutely still, afraid to move in case I dislodged what seemed to me to be masses of wire on top of my head. I felt they were attached to a battery and the words were going through my head."

Ena's wise advice to prospective sitters is that they can help to ensure good results by being open-minded and sympathetic during sittings to a medium's efforts to establish a bridge between two worlds. She says: "I don't mind if a person is drenched in grief. I can help them to control it and to relax. I don't ask them to trust me. All I ask is an unbiased approach. Very aggressive sitters create an impossible barrier. I also dislike sitters to interrogate me during a sitting. You can get into a muddle." Describing the onset of trance she says this begins with a sensation as if there were a blockage at the top of her spine around the back of her neck. "What I want to say is muzzy and won't come. I also become aware that I'm breathing deeply. Then I'm gone, and it is difficult to tell the precise moment when this happens."

Nan Mackenzie, on the other hand, describes trance as a "state of suspended animation". This gentle-voiced woman, a former hospital matron whose subsequent decades of dedicated trance healing—most of them associated with the Spiritualist Association of Great Britain—have won her countless friends, told me that at the onset of her trance condition she feels as though she were being gently and carefully withdrawn. "Sometimes I have the experience of looking down at my own body, but often I wake up with the remembrance of having been in a beautiful country-side." She never heals without prayer. She also believes no medium should ever go onto a platform without saying a prayer beforehand.

It can truly be said of her that she was born to heal, for even in the early arduous years of her hospital service she was able to establish an almost uncanny rapport with the sick and suffering. Indeed, on one occasion, the obdurate insistence of a patient who had refused to go into the operating theatre unless accompanied by the young probationer nurse with the heart-warming smile caused a strict hospital rule to be temporarily waived. In those days Nan Mackenzie knew little of psychic matters but she always accepted without questioning her puzzling power to have prevision of a patient's death. She says: "I knew nothing in those days of the etheric or astral body, but when a patient was dying I was always conscious of a 'presence' in the ward, often unseen but sometimes apparent in the form of a light mist." Her previsioning was not confined to deaths, for as a young nurse her talent as an amateur fortune-teller was in great demand among hospital colleagues and personal friends.

In her healing work, she is always entranced when making a diagnosis, but sometimes retains consciousness while giving healing. She is frank about her non-successes, saying: "Of course healing sometimes fails. It must be so, for otherwise no one would ever die. But even when it fails to restore health it takes away pain and so the person is able to pass quietly and simply into the spirit world."

Gerald Croiset, phenomenal Dutch clairvoyant whose unpaid help has frequently been enlisted to help solve difficult crimes, especially in locating missing children, has a particularly marked gift for breaking through time and space barriers and has told journalists: "The past, present and future are for me difficult to separate."

Croiset, whose telephone rarely stops ringing for long, becomes attentive when it happens to be a real call for help. At such times, he says, " a warning sensation disturbs me. I get a vibration like a full-up feeling and expand like a balloon. Then I know it is not an ordinary call." Frequently his clairvoyance is expressed in colours. "These," he says, "spin around in me very fast until they form a picture. The pictures shoot out as if they were flashing forward like a three-dimensional film." Fatigue tends to blur his clairvoyant images. Croiset tells us: "I have a gift from God which

I don't understand. I can't force it. I have to feel it is useful before I can help anybody. I don't use it just to make money for myself. If I do I may lose it."

Of Jewish parentage, Croiset has occasionally experienced visionary states in which angels have appeared to him but in general his psychic gifts do not appear to require the intervention of any "spirit" guardian or control. In his vivid biographical study *Croiset the Clairvoyant*, Jack Harrison Pollack also confirms that when the medium's "pictorial thinking" takes place the "twilight zone" withdrawal in Croiset can be so slight as to be scarcely noticeable to an observer.

Peter Hurkos, another world-famous Dutch psychic, whose talents manifested in 1943 after he had fractured his skull in a 30-feet fall from a painter's ladder, has also frequently helped police in investigations of difficult crimes.

In his autobiography *Psychic*, Hurkos, who regards his psychic talent as a very mixed blessing, has stated :

God has been kind to humanity, for if we could see all the impulses that travel through our atmosphere, we should soon go mad. Since we cannot see them, we forget that they exist. In my case, I am sensitive to a great degree even to these vibrations. I can shake hands with a person, and feel these emissions. I can also pick up these vibrations from an object a person has touched, from a piece of clothing he has worn, from a bed in which he has slept, from anything with which the person is associated, or even from a photograph of the person. . . . Every human also has a certain amount of the same psychic power I possess: mine is simply more developed. Most people do not use their gift.

He has also described what it is like to be on the receiving end of tests in a Faraday cage in an American parapsychologist's laboratory—in this case that of Dr Andrija Puharich. The doctor had explained to him that the object of the isolated, insulated cubicle, covered outside by a fine copper mesh, through which a generator poured 250,000 volts of electric current, was to set up an electrical field through which no electrical waves could pass. It took days of persuasion before Hurkos could overcome his fear of entering the cage.

At best the Faraday cage was a nerve-wracking experience. I could not stay inside for more than an hour without feeling as though I were strangling. The air got hot and foul, and every unaccustomed noise made me believe something had gone wrong and I could never come out alive. Even with Dr Puharich inside, as he was in the beginning, I was nervous. Sometimes I thought I could not draw another breath.

... The strange thing I found when I was inside the cage and the current roared, was that my powers were greater than ever inside this electrical field, isolated from the normal disturbance of the atmosphere. I did better in all the usual tests than I had ever done before.

Confirming the extreme fear of electricity experienced by Peter Hurkos, Dr Puharich has expressed the view that this probably helped to ensure the excellence of test results, because, in research terminology, it induced a "true crisis adrenergia based on a feeling of flight, fright, or fight." It is well known that spontaneous telepathy and other psychic phenomena takes place in conditions of fear, crisis, or extreme danger and Puharich has described in *Beyond Telepathy* an experiment which appears to bear this out.

Under normal test conditions he had found that Hurkos, as a telepathic sender working with another sensitive under normal room conditions, achieved only average scores of about 12 hits out of 50 ESP-test trials. Puharich therefore devised an experiment which necessitated Hurkos actually sitting on a foot plate which had a ten-thousand-volt direct current charge on it. Puharich tells us:

Actually the nature of the charge was such that even though Hurkos was sitting on the foot plate and the electricity was turned on, he would not experience any shock. I explained this carefully to Peter and assured him that he would not in any way be hurt. He was enterprising enough to go ahead with the experiment, but I could see grave doubts and fears written all over his face as the experiment began. The experiment was extraordinarily successful. The average score jumped from the twelve correct hits out of fifty to thirty-one correct hits out of fifty trials. This is overwhelming evidence of telepathic inter-action. There was no doubt that Hurkos' fear was profound as he sat on the electrically charged foot plate. I repeated these experiments seven times with the same results.

Summing up his own manifold experiences with outstanding mediums Puharich states: "It is difficult to escape the conclusion that mind at certain levels of operation is ubiquitous and can pass through the barriers of the physical world around us. In fact there are times when it literally transcends time as it leaps ahead to cognize physical events not yet born, or leaps backwards in time to reconstruct scenes long since perished from the physical realm."

4. Geraldine Cummins

CUMMINS, Geraldine Dorothy: Author. Daughter of late Prof. Ashley Cummins, M.D. and Jane Constable. Educ. home. Publications: The Land They Loved, Fires of Beltane, Irish novels; Variety Show (short stories); The Scripts of Cleophas; Paul in Athens; The Great Days of Ephesus; The Childhood of Jesus; Beyond Human Personality; The Road to Immortality; They Survive (with E. B. Gibbes); When Nero Was Dictator; After Pentecost; Healing the Mind (with Dr Connell); Travellers in Eternity; I Appeal Unto Caesar; The Manhood of Jesus; D. E. Œ. Somerville (biography); Unseen Adventures (autobiographical); The Fate of Colonel Fawcett; Mind in Life and Death; Swan on a Black Sea; plays produced: Till Yesterday Comes Again; three Irish Plays (with S. R. Day): Broken Faith, Fox and Geese, The Way of the World; two books translated into 4 languages; has contributed short stories or articles to periodicals and magazines. Recreations: gardening, tennis, music, played in the Irish International Hockey Team. . . .

As a potted professional biography the above entry in *Who's Who* at the time of Geraldine Cummins' death on August 24, 1969, can hardly be bettered, yet, unwittingly, it conveys a ludicrously misleading impression.

The innocent reader will promptly picture a daunting, athletic bluestocking endowed with a voracious appetite for historical research of a strongly religious and polemical bent; possessor of a vigorous self-confidence and a surplus of physical and mental energy which spills over into a fiercely nationalistic flood of novels, plays, stories and articles leavened by sportive forays on hard courts and hockey fields.

Nothing could be further from the truth. Incurably shy and self-effacing, this diminutive, twinkling-eyed septuagenarian cherished a lifelong aversion to the academic and pretentious. Wiry and courageous, but possessed of a deceptively frail physique, she regarded herself as under-vitalized, and was always so far removed from any pretentions to literary punditry that she insisted on proclaiming that she had "not composed a single sentence" of many of the books which—rightly—carry her name on the title pages. To cap all, she had long lived in such scholarly seclusion that her closest neighbours in London and even in Ireland, where she spent up to six months of each year, would probably be among the most surprised to learn that she had ever put public pen to paper. Indeed she belonged by nature, choice and unusual gifts, to that increasingly rare category of human beings who can with truth be described as having in their lifetimes walked backwards into fame not of their seeking, in fields not of their primary choice.

Yet, if the Greater London Council continues its present endearing practice of publicizing the homes of former distinguished residents, then a certain three-storey house of indeterminate architecture in a quiet street off King's Road, Chelsea, may well one day display a blue wall plaque proclaiming: *Geraldine Cummins Lived Here....*

And the more perceptive among those who in years to come may visit this unobtrusive thoroughfare to pay posthumous passing homage to Chelsea's former seeress of the pen, will note a characteristic minor irony of history. Mid-twentieth-century Chelsea takes pride in its reputation as an internationally-famed haunt for artists and avant-garde intelligentsia. The presence, however, for 35 years in their midst of a shy, witty woman whom Prime Ministers, scientists and philosophers considered themselves privileged to consult in arcane matters, passed virtually unnoticed. True, in 1966, on one notable occasion at which I myself was in attendance in a professional capacity, her home was invaded by a lively team of television experts to record her at her literary and uncanny labours. But, again, it is significant that the first television tribute came from across the Atlantic, not from the islands in which she was born and spent a lifetime.

Fifth child in a family of eleven, sired by an overworked, warm-hearted Professor of Medicine popularly nicknamed the

"Poor Man's Doctor", Geraldine was born in a Georgian house in St Patrick's Square by the banks of the River Lee in rebel Cork.

She inherited not only her father's humanism and his Celtic blue-grey eyes, but also his insatiable intellectual curiosity as to the nature of those "physiological and psychological units" we term human beings. Her mother was opposed to her youthful wish to follow in her father's professional footsteps so Geraldine with some reluctance eventually opted for the pen instead of the desired scalpel.

And this dreaming, tomboy girl—always happiest in the rural retreat, aptly named Woodville, which again became the family home after a lapse of generations—proved an apt aspirant in the literary field. At the early age of 22 she experienced what she has described as "the youthful bliss" of having one of her first plays, *Broken Faith* (written in collaboration with a friend, Susanne Day), put on at Dublin's Abbey Theatre, under the auspicious joint direction of W. B. Yeats and Lennox Robinson.

Soon she was having her short stories published by London's *Pall Mall Gazette* and all seemed set for a conventionally successful literary career. But three fateful encounters in her twenties set her questing in a very unforeseen direction: amateur mediumship, in the unlikely form of "transmitted writing", popularly, but less accurately described as "automatic writing".

In her own sparkling autobiography, *Unseen Adventures*, Geraldine has told how her childish interest in ghosts was re-kindled through her first meeting with Mrs Hester Dowden, imperious, talented daughter of a famous Irish Shakespearian scholar, Professor Edward Dowden. Hester Dowden's own considerable psychic powers had earlier impressed Sir Oliver Lodge, the famous physicist who became an indefatigable pioneer psychic researcher.

It was during a holiday in Paris, while staying at the Hotel Normandie, that Geraldine first encountered the formidable Hester, and attended her first seance :

While thunder pealed and the room darkened I was suitably thrilled by Mrs Dowden's demonstration of her psychic powers. There were no eerie, visible manifestations. At that time Mrs Dowden obtained messages from alleged deceased persons on the ouija-board. It is a sheet of cardboard on which the letters of the alphabet are printed. The automatist's fingers rest on a small heart-shaped piece of polished wood called a "traveller" or "pointer". This "traveller" glides lightly over the cardboard pointing to the letters spelling out messages.

The first communication on this occasion came from Mrs Dowden's daemon or control Eyen. He soon introduced a deceased Frenchman, some of whose remarks were decidedly sensational. He said "rivers of blood will flow in France." He prophesied that "many houses will be destroyed, great numbers of people rendered homeless and thousands will die." He was not given an opportunity to state in what way these horrors would be accomplished. For, before any further details were conveyed, Mrs Dowden took her hand off the "traveller" and airily remarked that her communicators quite frequently told lies, and she did not believe a word of this prophecy. She made me from that moment extremely critical in my analysis of subsequent messages. It is an excellent habit in a medium.

Nevertheless that seance understandably left an indelible impression, for the date of the sitting was June 1914. And Geraldine's literary fate, in the sense of an eventual major switch away from exclusive concentration on fictional writing towards the increasingly intensive participation in controlled psychic experiments with "transmitted" factual scripts which eventually brought her international fame among researchers, may be said to have been sealed when she took a wartime job cataloguing eighteenth-century sermons in Dublin's National Library and became a paying guest in Mrs Dowden's home in Lower Fitzwilliam Street.

In Mrs Dowden's social circle musical evenings were frequently interspersed with psychic experiments. Under her tuition Geraldine began to get messages on the ouija board. Her apprenticeship as an amateur medium was to prove prolonged. She has frankly stated : "I had no spontaneous psychic experiences during my childhood. I have trained myself to be a medium and years of hard, often dull, work of the plodding laboratory type were necessary for this development."

Her first attempt to obtain a psychic message was made with Lennox Robinson, the Irish playwright : "He and I sat at the ouija board for nearly an hour and obtained only three words—'Pruss under water.' This illuminating seance only whetted my appetite for more." But she long remained sceptical, attributing any subsequent "hits" to a co-operative subconscious.

Second fateful encounter in that Dublin period of her career was a meeting with the benign poet and mystic, A. E. (George Russell), who gave her wise counsel on Eastern exercises to develop inner detachment: "Briefly A. E. advised concentrating intently on an object such as a 'White Triangle', or on a single word, for at first a very few minutes, three or four perhaps, as the whole attention had to be uninterruptingly fixed on the object with every stray thought eliminated. Some years later, when I had begun psychic experiments, I carried out this advice. I chose the word 'stillness', perceiving it meditatively in my mind's eye, for a few minutes only, while I endeavoured to lose my little self in the meaning of that word."

As her mediumship developed there emerged what she has described as "an amplification of A. E.'s advice, a response perhaps from the Unknown to my request for aid in an apparently impossible task."

The "impossible task" to which she referred was connected with a "test" sitting given in 1925 in the study of the late Dr Maude, Bishop of Kensington, in the presence of several scholars, including a well-known Hebrew scholar, the late Prebendary W. O. E. Oesterley, D.D., Emeritus Professor of Hebrew and Old Testament Exegesis in King's College, London University. They had foregathered to witness Geraldine write down one of her transmitted scripts, eventually published in a series of books collectively known as *The Scripts of Cleophas*. These comprised evidential accounts of early Christian history and the transmitted writings eventually totalled over a million words. Geraldine knew neither Greek, Hebrew nor Latin. Her reading had been confined mainly to modern literature, yet Dr Oesterley and other named scholars have testified that the Cleophas scripts "contain much which, on consideration of the life and mentality of the inter-mediary, Miss Cummins, appears quite inexplicable on the supposition of human authorship."

Obtained at intervals in the twenties and thirties, the scripts were not only frequently written in the presence of learned witnesses, but throughout were also supervised, checked and edited by an English researcher, Miss E. B. Gibbes, a member of the Society for Psychical Research. Beatrice Gibbes and Geraldine first met in 1923. It proved a pregnant, path-changing event. They became friends and collaborated in a twenty-year research partnership about which Geraldine later wrote :

> Representatives of the Society for Psychical Research have complained that mediums will not work for the Society. But, in one sense, I have done so for 20 years in the best way possible. I gave sittings to six of the Society's presidents and also almost continuously to E. B. G. Being a member of the S.P.R. she employed the thorough and exhaustive methods of investigation for which this Society is renowned. But, in one respect, she went further than any other representative of it, as she kept her laboratory specimen (myself) under observation in her house, with the exception of holidays, over a period of 20 years.

But I stray. To return to the worthy Dr Maude. Geraldine has confessed that in those still early days of her mind-experimenting, the Bishop's invitation aroused "extreme fear and tension. . . . The experiment seemed doomed to failure. These Cleophas scripts were of a period in early Christian history of which I was totally ignorant, so I had no idea beforehand what would be written. My conscious mind was helpless in the matter."

In the solitude of her room a few days before the experiment she tells us that "advice" was somehow transmitted to her that in the quiet of evening she should do three things. First she must concentrate on stillness; second on her desire that in the Bishop's study the pen she held would move rapidly and well—and finally, she must imagine her desire has been fulfilled.

In an illuminating passage she describes the process as follows :

> In order to enter the stillness, it is necessary to raise one's intelligence to a higher degree of consciousness. The stillness is neither a passive, inert state, nor trance, in my experience. When achieved it is a lucid work of intense activity. The condition of stillness clarifies the desire and creates efficiency. Once launched, the desire seems as a little boat on the lake or sea of the imagination. There, piloted by desire, driven forward by the waves of imagination, it can on certain occasions reach the objective chosen.

When the day of the ordeal arrived she achieved success, thanks to her nights of preparation. Seated at the table with virgin foolscap sheets before her she shaded her eyes with one hand while the other held the pen. A tranquillity descended upon her and for an hour and a half, oblivious of a thunderstorm raging outside and of the seven watchful critics, she completed a ten folio chapter of historical narrative without a pause. It comprises chapter 30 of *The Scripts of Cleophas*.

This rapidity of writing is an outstanding supernormal feature of Geraldine's transmitted scripts, whether they concern historical material or survival communications. In her transmitted writing a speed of up to 2000 words an *hour* has frequently been attested, yet in normal writing she works slowly and laboriously.

A fellow author and psychic researcher, Signe Toksvig, who meticulously edited the "Black Swan" scripts obtained by Geraldine, has said of her mediumship: "Not since Swedenborg, it seems to me, has there been so absorbing a case of double authorship, of one who is able to function on both sides of the curtain while still in the flesh." Mme Toksvig can speak with authority for her own interest in psychic matters was first aroused when she was making preparatory studies for her praised biography of Emanuel Swedenborg, eighteenth-century Swedish scientist and mystic.

Swedenborg, she tells us, confessed in his diaries that at times his hand seemed to write "of itself" often, as in the case of Geraldine Cummins, things with which he disagreed.

In the case of the Cleophas scripts they were said to have been "dictated" to the medium by a "Group of Seven Messengers". And it is of interest that William Blake, England's poet-artist mystic, has also stated that he too wrote "under the direction of Messengers daily and nightly". His prophetical book *Jerusalem*, he has affirmed, "was written from immediate dictation, twelve or sometimes twenty or thirty lines at a time, without premeditation and even against my will." In a letter written on April 25, 1803, to Thomas Butts he stated: "I have written this poem ('Milton') from immediate dictation. I can praise it since I dare not pretend to be any other than the secretary; the authors are in Eternity."

Geraldine was never dogmatic about the possible source of her transmitted or inspirational, factually evidential scripts, she merely tells us that in the case of taking down the Cleophas scripts she was "in an almost completely dream state" and believed she was possibly operating on a superconscious level.

It is a fascinating fact that her first experiment in "entering into the stillness" occurred at an early sitting given in Hester Dowden's home to the poet W. B. Yeats. The results were recorded by this imperious lady who grew impatient when her young pupil began to describe, in poetic language, a "thrilling narrative about an ancient castle in the west of Ireland and dramatic events that took place in it to a family living there." Hester suddenly stopped Geraldine's ouija board performance, saying: "Mr Yeats, this is a story, but there is no communicator, so it is not of interest." Yeats did not agree. "On the contrary," he told his surprised hostess, "I find it of intense interest as it is exactly the plot and drama of the play I am at present writing, and so far I have told it to no one."

On the face of it this would seem a classic instance of a medium having obtained her information by means of telepathy or clairvoyance from Yeats. Yeats obviously thought so, too, for he immediately embarked upon a telepathic experiment. Successively he mentally concentrated upon five different objects and pictures in the room. The medium did not succeed in getting any correct. Her own theory is that when W. B. Yeats was composing his drama he was "physically living on the superconscious level of an advanced mind life. His presence then enabled me to rise to that level and to record it on the superconscious level, uttering aloud in his poetic language the narrative of this drama and his new play."

Certainly it requires an infinite stretching of the telepathic theory to account for those by no means infrequent instances in Survival proofs when Geraldine's psychic powers obtained verified "facts that nobody knows", some of them prophetic. To quote just one of many striking instances: In the first script written by Geraldine for Mackenzie King, the Canadian Premier, the communicator, Roosevelt, foresaw the unexpected outbreak of the Korean War two years later and also predicted De Gaulle's coming to power in France 11 years later.

Her first two personally shattering experiences of previsioning occurred during World War 1, when she foresaw in sleep the precise circumstances of the front line deaths of two officer brothers. In the case of her brother Harry, killed in Gallipoli, the veridical dream occurred several days before the tragedy. Similarly, her dream about the death of her brother Fenton in France took place 17 days before the event. Fellow officers later confirmed the accuracy of Geraldine's tragic previsioning.

CROWNING TRIUMPH

For many years Geraldine's mediumship has attracted interest and increasing respect from leading researchers. A reviewer in the *Journal of the Society for Psychical Research* said of her first book of published scripts (*They Survive*) that they provided remarkable evidence of "genuineness and outstanding quality". Praising "the high standard of accuracy evidenced" the critic recommended it as well worth study by "any person with a scientific mind and no strong prejudice".

Her crowning research achievement,* undertaken at the request of Mr W. H. Salter, a veteran researcher who for many years was honorary secretary of the Society for Psychical Research, happened in the evening of her mediumship.

This great adventure of the mind began unexpectedly when she was on holiday in Bantry Bay, in August, 1957. Salter had sent her a letter containing a very strange request. "A member of the S.P.R. who lost his mother some months ago would like to give her the opportunity of sending him a message. I believe that this is a case that would interest you evidentially; ... I should propose to restrict the information given you to the name of 'the absent sitter', so as to make a success all the more striking." The challenge was accepted and the momentous two-worlds weaving of a psychic masterpiece began. Never was any woman set a seemingly more impossible task!

Equipped solely with the gossamer armoury of the name of a man unknown to her, Major Henry Tennant, she had been bidden to cast her psychic net beyond the earth's boundaries and to quest among the myriad "dead" for a stranger. The "mad Irish" are famed for intrepidity. Though Geraldine was offered the additional help of specimens of the "dead" woman's handwriting, she adhered to the basic principle long honoured by the most adventurous pioneers—"In for a penny, in for a pound." She tells us, "Owing to my capacity for object reading, I preferred to

* *Swan on a Black Sea* by Geraldine Cummins.

61

try without the specimens of the mother's handwriting, and the first three scripts were obtained by me without them." It should also be noted that *all* the eventual forty published scripts were obtained when she was alone, "in most instances in the bright light of the early morning before I had met anybody".

Unknown to Geraldine, Major Henry Tennant was the youngest son of Mrs Charles Coombe Tennant. During her lifetime her mediumistic gifts had been kept a strictly guarded secret, even from her own sons who never suspected that she was the famous "Mrs Willett" whose psychic gifts at the turn of the century had played so important a part in probably the most remarkable experiment ever undertaken in Western psychic research. This experiment—famed as the S.P.R.'s unchallenged "Cross-Correspondence Case"—began in 1901, following Frederic Myers' death, and continued until 1930. It involved well over 3,000 scripts purporting to come from the surviving spirits of Myers and other founders of the S.P.R., and involved the separate efforts of a remarkable group of about a dozen "automatists", only one of whom (Mrs Piper) was a professional medium.

Geraldine knew no member or friend of the Coombe Tennant family and she did not meet either of "Mrs Willett's" surviving sons until after the fortieth script had been written on November 23, 1959.

While it is the copious, meticulously researched "evidence" which will increasingly continue to impress investigators, it is the impetuous, sparkling personality of the "communicator" which is likely to make a lasting impress on the general reader for "Mrs Willett" survives as the formidable, fascinating personality she was reputed to be in her lifetime.

A skilled society hostess and devoted mother, she became Britain's first woman magistrate and first woman delegate to the League of Nations.

Verbally she explodes in every script, true to, but *larger* than life. Not surprisingly, it wasn't long before the communicator's sceptical son Henry, who received the scripts by post, wrote to Miss Cummins. "The more I study these scripts the more deeply I am impressed by them." He confirmed that with the exception of one incorrect name, "every other name and reference is accurate and to me very evidential and at times surprising. *There was no tapping of my mind because much appears that I never knew.*"

In his first letter to Geraldine, Henry Tennant confessed that he was an atheist. The effect of this revelation upon his mother was dramatic. The transmitted writing became violently agitated as the "mother" replied :

The magistrate is the prisoner in the dock, and her son is judge and jury. He has to give a verdict in an unusual law case. There is, I think, no precedent. At any rate no magistrate was ever tried before in a law court with her son as a judge to decide the issue. Briefly, what is the issue, my Lord? Does the prisoner exist or does she not?

The scripts which give her "case for the defence" are unique in psychic literature for this "quick-silvered" woman presents her manifold arguments and evidence with characteristic humour and irony. At the end of her plea she tells her son, "My Lord, you may sentence the mother to annihilation, but for the son somewhere is buried the uneasy suspicion that a fragment of her goes on living and loving him." Posthumously lifting her lifelong ban on personal publicity "Mrs Willett" also transmitted a message to Salter :

Dear W. H., I lift my ban entirely. . . . There comes to me from the earth such a feeling or impression, of worrying, of anxiety, of fear of death, and it is derived from non-belief. If they could but realize half the glory, even a fragment of the peace of this life I now experience.
    If I could only make them accept it, there might at least be some rationality. Rationalists are irrational, and it makes such a confusion, creates so much fear, when death, that deliverer, approaches.
Dear Death.
Yours, Win.

Understandably publication of the forty "Willett" scripts in 1965 created a furore of excitement and praise among Western psychic researchers, who included three former presidents of the S.P.R., headed by Salter. At an early stage in the apparently impossible experiment he had become impressed by their veridical content. At one point when Geraldine had almost decided to discontinue the scripts, he told her: "Your scripts are among the most interesting developments in psychical research for many years."

Similarly, after publication, Dr R. H. Thouless, a Fellow of Corpus Christi College, Cambridge, another ex-President of the S.P.R., described the scripts as ". . . the strongest evidence for a real communicator that I have ever seen. It shows, I think, the great gifts of Geraldine Cummins as a medium (or interpreter) although its success may also be attributed to the unique gifts of Mrs Tennant as a communicator."

And the major research tribute to this survival testament is expressed in a 52-page, documented foreword written by a third former S.P.R. President, Professor C. D. Broad, Fellow of Trinity College, Cambridge. "I believe," he writes, "that these automatic scripts are a very important addition to the vast mass of such material which *prima facie* suggests rather strongly that certain human beings have survived the death of their physical bodies and have been able to communicate with certain others who are still in the flesh."

His testimony is the more striking because, though he had never met Geraldine, or the Danish editor, Signe Toksvig, he reveals that Major Henry Tennant—to whom the scripts are addressed— had been his pupil at Cambridge and had later become a lifelong friend.

Broad points out that the scripts abound in extremely concrete detail about named persons and places, and about definite events in which these were concerned. "Moreover, of the large mass of concrete testable statements, very nearly all are true. When a mistake is made . . . it is nearly always corrected in a later script."

He bluntly adds: "Obviously much the simplest and most plausible hypothesis *prima facie* is that Mrs Coombe Tennant, or some aspect of her, survived the death of her body on August 31, 1956; that she was still actively in existence at least as late as March 6, 1960; and that during that period she from time to time controlled, directly or indirectly, the pen of the automatist G. C."

With characteristic academic thoroughness he explores two "conceivable alternatives", including what he describes as "the fantastic hypothesis, involving telepathy and clairvoyance on the part of those still in the flesh." He dryly concludes by inviting readers "to study carefully for themselves the scripts and the notes on them, and to draw their own conclusions as to what is, rather literally, a 'question of life or death'."

Geraldine's little known co-partnership with her brother Robert, a Cork physician, in a remarkable series of psycho-medical investigations carried out at intervals over a period of some twenty years, has been described by him in a book titled *Healing the Mind* published under the protective pseudonym of R. Connell M.D. It posed the question : Can the little explored faculty of the mind popularly termed ESP (extra-sensory perception) be utilized effectively in the investigation and treatment of baffling psychoses? These published case histories provide an affirmative answer.

I can personally testify that the doctor-author, whom I was privileged to meet and come to know well in the later years of his retirement, is an outstanding example of dedicated professionalism. Throughout his long professional life he was always courageously loyal to the conviction that it must always be the primary aim of a family doctor to cure his patient even if, as in the cases described, it involved going a step beyond conventionally accepted medical techniques.

In his foreword to the above-mentioned book he has frankly acknowledged the major collaborative help given by Geraldine whose aid he had successfully sought in each of the described case histories. He tells us: "To her expert and highly trained mind much of the success achieved can be ascribed." He has also emphasized the duty of a doctor to pursue his healing objective, even if he does not fully understand the method or weapon he employs, or how it achieves its purpose :

Research into these aspects is incidental. The family physician has not been engaged in proving any scientific hypothesis in regard to ESP, or in investigating the ranges of the conscious and subconscious human mind. The object has been to cure or relieve his patients. Exact scientific observation and proofs of the sensitive's findings, have not been pursued beyond the needs of the case in consequence, and any deductions made are therefore limited.

Dr Connell also makes it plain that in each of the cases described his unorthodox researches, aided by "the services of an unusually expert sensitive", were undertaken in the interests of the patient concerned only after the available resources of medicine, including specialists and psychoanalysts, had proved ineffectual.

His first "adventure" concerned a tragic case of protracted bouts of intermittent alcoholism associated with a writing inhibition. The patient had twice undergone courses of treatment in nursing homes and had suffered relapses, but the doctor's interest had been aroused by the fact that repeatedly—on at least six occasions—the patient had been able, temporarily at least, to abstain entirely from drinking. When he pressed the patient as to why he did not forswear excessive drinking permanently he was told : "It is not the alcohol—for it I care nothing—but I must confess I discovered after my father's death that on certain occasions—when, I never knew—I found I could not sign my name. An employee would bring half a dozen cheques to sign, possibly trivial; it would not matter. I would take up my pen; it would be impossible. At other times I could sign readily. I never knew . . . I discovered that a dose of alcohol would overcome the inhibition."

When the patient also revealed that he appeared to be suffering from an *inherited* writing inhibition—his father had been forced to retire from the chairmanship of the firm because of the same psychotic disability—Dr Connell became anxious. The psychosis obviously had its roots in a race heritage since it had been handed down from father to son. The man's plight was acute and psychiatrists had repeatedly failed to track down the cause.

Dr Connell decided to enlist the help of ESP in an endeavour to trace the historic cause of the writing inhibition. He borrowed from the patient an old family document relating how the Freedom of the City of London had been conferred on two of the patient's ancestors in the years 1731 and 1762 respectively.

This document was sent to Miss Cummins who was asked to report upon it, using her psychic gift for object-reading. This process is known as psychometry and it is explained by Dr Connell as follows :

It has been known for many years that if an object belonging to an individual is submitted to an adept in ESP, that is a person who has practised and developed this faculty of the mind of which we speak, then the adept is capable of giving a very accurate account of the character of the owner, or past owner, of events in his life and past history, and even events of significance in the lives of ancestors in a similar pattern. These accounts are individual, their truth cannot always be vouched for, save by inference, or on occasion sometimes by historic research. They are not limited by time or space.

Geraldine's report revealed that the patient had inherited a deep family fear generated by a terrible act of persecution enacted by the Inquisition in Spain. She reported that the family's race name in Spain had been Davila, a fact subsequently checked and verified. An eldest son of the family had married a woman of the Spanish nobility and letters written by her had fallen into the hands of the Inquisition. Every member of the family was seized, including the husband who died under torture, cursing his wife who had been forced to witness his sufferings on the rack and wheel. She was carrying her first child, a son, born while she was insane. The Report stated that the unhappy woman had found herself unable ever again to write; when her escape to London was finally achieved she prohibited her son ever to attempt to write. Many facts in Geraldine's object reading were later verified, and the writing inhibition was discovered to have affected at least nine members in varying branches of the family.

Most important of all, the cathartic shock impact of the revealed family history led to the final cure of the patient. He recovered completely from the writing inhibition. There were only two minor relapses over a long period of years and he achieved additional business success, becoming chairman of the company.

Another successful and striking case—subject of a later medical lecture in Cork—concerned the successful treatment, using ESP, of a 50-year-old architect who had become totally incapacitated for $8\frac{1}{2}$ years with violent pains in his legs and neck. When Dr Connell was brought in to the case the unfortunate man, his career in ruins, had consulted five practitioners (two professors, two psychiatrists and a practitioner of hypnotism) whose services had proved unavailing in alleviating his physical torment. The physical nervous system had been pronounced perfectly sound.

The patient's fountain pen was borrowed and despatched to

Geraldine in London and the eventual "report" indicated that the patient's mind-illness, or psychosis, had been engendered through the folly of a young nursemaid who had left the three-year-old boy unattended. During her absence a piece of furniture had fallen on the child pinioning him by the legs and neck. When she returned the nurse had frightened the child with threats if he revealed what had happened to his parents. It was the beginning of a fear complex, later enhanced when his father was fatally injured in lifting too heavy a load. Other associated family tragedies were also correctly indicated. Her findings were explained to the patient and the resulting improvement in his condition was sustained. He was encouraged to take advantage of an opportunity to take up an endowed course at an English University and he eventually became the successful Unitarian minister of a large parish.

In his book, and in a later lecture to fellow doctors, Dr Connell described the case histories as a form of "abreactive therapy" by means of which the dramatic portrayal of the psychically discovered cause of the psychosis leads to its disappearance and the recovery of the patient affected.

He pointed out that "abreactive therapy" had become an increasingly effective medical technique in the Second World War and afterwards, and referred to William Sargant's *Battle for the Mind* which describes how over 1,000 patients were effectively treated by this type of therapy. In these war cases, however, the violent experiences of fear that initiated the mental illness were neither obscure nor distant. Many psychoses are more complex and of longer duration and Dr Connell rightly points out that few patients have either the time or the financial means to submit to protracted psychoanalytic treatment which may last up to two or three years. It is in the treatment of such complex psychoses, sometimes necessitating a probing of family and even racial history, that he believes the tool of ESP, properly used, could be of great value to the psychoanalyst.

By short circuiting his investigations it would enable him to concentrate on his essential work, that of resynthesizing the personality of his patient, and of preventing any return of the emotional complex after its disclosure and resolution. The strengthening, fortifying and building up of the personality of his patient are essential after the crisis he has passed through.

The method of recovering race memories by free association, and by deductions from symbolic dreams, must be, by its very nature, a somewhat tedious and prolonged research. ESP appears to be the only other method of obtaining the race history in a single interview or its equivalent. Even deep hypnosis does not probe beyond the individual life.

And dreaming into the future the author predicted a practical role for ESP in psychological medicine, if potentially gifted sensitives could be carefully selected and trained. He suggests that the Department of Psychology in a university could be the proper authority to back such an innovation. "It is their duty and purpose," he says, "to investigate the range of the human mind. ESP in all its aspects appertains to the mind and is essentially their work." He believes that use of sensitives, effectively controlled and financially supported, could in time prove of the greatest value not only in medicine but also in other fields of scientific and intellectual research. It is an idea which should not be too lightly dismissed.

5. Surgeon in Two Worlds

One of my most way-out assignments in journalism led me on a November afternoon in 1963 to the pleasant market town of Aylesbury to inquire a little further into the stranger-than-fiction experience of a Mrs Ethel J. Bailey, of Streatham Hill, London.

The lady claimed that very recently she had shaken hands and chatted to a well-known optical surgeon-consultant who had *died* 26 years earlier. She had last seen Dr Lang alive 48 years ago in Moorfields Eye Hospital when she had consulted him on the advisability of an operation on a "lazy" eye and a permanently closed right eyelid. Furthermore, she now declared that as a result of her 1963 encounter with the "dead" surgeon her eyelid trouble had vanished and she had also begun to see better with the right eye.

Was Mrs Bailey mad or suffering from hallucinatory delusions? Yet apart from her seemingly "impossible" claims she appeared to be robustly normal in the fullest sense of the word.

She had told how on that earlier occasion Lang had been characteristically kindly but blunt. "Yes," he had told the 21-year-old girl's mother. "The operation *could* be performed but the unsatisfactory result would be that the eyelid would then be pinned permanently open." The young woman's fiancé had also advised against it and the operation was never performed.

Many years passed. Mrs Bailey eventually married, brought up a family, and in her later years had become interested in Spiritualism and spirit healing. One day in her late sixties she had been startled to read about a "Dr Lang" who was reported to be achieving remarkable healing results as the "spirit" control of a former Aylesbury fireman, Mr George Chapman.

At first she presumed that the "Dr Lang" referred to in newspaper reports must be Cosmo Lang, a former Archbishop of

Canterbury. Then she idly wondered whether he might possibly be a relative of "*my* Mr Lang from Moorfields". Curiosity nagged; finally she had made up her mind to write to George Chapman for an appointment. When she was taken into the "surgery" to meet "Mr Lang", who spoke to her through the body of the entranced medium, recognition, it appeared, had been "mutual and instantaneous".

"Lang," she said, "appeared exactly as I remembered him so far as his mannerisms were concerned. It was definitely the same Lang. And he recognized me, too." Smilingly he had reminded her that when she last visited him she had only weighed about seven stones. Mrs Bailey, who had grown more buxom with middle age, had agreed he wouldn't be far out in his estimate.

Lang, she related, had then told her to lie on his healing couch so that he could perform—on her "spirit" or "Etheric" body—the long-postponed operation to rectify the muscular deficiency in her closed right eyelid.

At the time of my own visit to Aylesbury Mrs Bailey had already reported that as a result of that "spirit" operation she had begun to be able to blink her right eyelid. Furthermore, she had also begun to have restored vision in her right eye.

When I, in my turn, had the strange privilege of meeting and questioning the "dead" surgeon in his posthumous Aylesbury "surgery", I asked him if he remembered Mrs Bailey's visit.

"Of course I do", he replied. "I also remember she was so thin when she first came to see me at Moorfields years ago I had advised her parents to give her malt."

"Do you remember many of your earthly patients?"

"I remember them all", he said. "Why, only the other day I spotted an eye scar on a patient. It was the sequel to an operation I had performed in the 1880's at the Middlesex Hospital when she had been only two years old." Laughing heartily he confessed: "I recognized my bad sewing. My colleagues used to tell me, 'Lang, you ought to get a young nurse to do your patching up'."

Then it was *my* turn to be surprised—like many hundreds of other Aylesbury patients—by a display of the "spirit" surgeon's astonishing diagnostic skill. As I have mentioned in another chapter, I have suffered most of my life from bronchiectasis, or dilation of the bronchial tubes. When Lang unexpectedly invited me to place myself on the surgery couch, for an examination and "spirit" operation, he swiftly diagnosed the lung condition which my own family doctor had failed to detect, explaining in medical terms the precise area of the trouble and the reason why an eventual operation had not been deemed practicable. He also correctly diagnosed an associated heart strain symptom of recent development about which I had told no-one. I can say now, with deep gratitude both to George Chapman and William Lang, that my unexpected and painless "operation" on that November afternoon brought me considerable easement and led to an eventual cessation of sporadic attacks of bronchial asthma which had become a troublesome side-effect of my illness.

I also recall that on that first occasion Lang also expressed the view that "mediums are born, and that's the top and bottom of it". He stressed, "There are many doctors on this side who want to return and work through ordinary, unselfish chaps like George." The difficulty, he added, a little sadly, was finding suitable human channels.

Patients privileged to receive the continued services of this formerly famous London surgeon, are likely to concur on two important aspects of the Chapman-Lang healing partnership.

First, the astonishing physical and personality differences which abundantly testify to the completeness of Lang's control of George Chapman during trance. George Chapman, still in his forties, was only 16 when Lang died at the age of 84. Mannerisms, medical knowledge, speech and gestures are startlingly contrasted.

Secondly, the "reality" of the "spirit" takeover is also manifested for many patients, including myself, in the extraordinary feeling of comfort and exhilaration experienced during treatment from the "spirit" surgeon. This aspect is admirably summed-up in a tribute given by one of Lang's patients, Mrs A. Farrelly, of Park Road, Kingston, Surrey. Praising the benefit she had received through Lang's ministrations, after her own doctor had told her nothing more could be done to bring back power in her right leg, she has testified:

I felt very uplifted after my visit. I felt I had been talking to an angel, which, of course, I had. It is eight or nine weeks since I went to Aylesbury. I can now put my leg up and down quite easily, cross one leg over the other and go upstairs again.

It is little wonder that every postman in the Aylesbury area knows the address of the Chapman home. Appeals for treatment appointments or absent healing reach this medium from all over the world. He receives upwards of 1,500 letters a week and it is the one expressed pride of this modest, big-hearted medium that no appeal goes unacknowledged.

Chapman's working day begins at 7.30 when he begins to open the massive daily post. An hour later, before the arrival of the office team, he has already begun to record replies into a dictating machine.

By noon Chapman and his devoted wife Margaret, who acts as receptionist, are ready to meet the first patients arriving for the daily week-day trance session which can last up to six-hours. I myself was present during a six-hour trance session which I witnessed in January, 1966, on the ground-floor of a house in Silver Street, Birmingham 14.

At the time of my memorable visit, Birmingham's most remarkable "clinic" had been established nearly ten years. The house bore no doctor's name-plate to distinguish it from its neighbours in the narrow street of old-fashioned terrace-type houses. It didn't need one for the ever-spreading fame of its visiting "spirit surgeon" filled it month after month with eager patients from all parts of the city and surrounding Midland counties. They arrived on foot, by bicycle, car, wheel-chair, train and mini-bus, packing the cheerful waiting room and sometimes overflowing through a spotless kitchen-scullery into the rear yard.

On the day of my visit the first twenty visitors to arrive by 11 a.m.—there were over seventy patients that day—had arrived by minibus from Manchester after a nearly four-hour journey through snow and sleet. This group's lively organizer, Mrs May Perry from Chorlton, told me she had formerly been a state nurse, and owed her life to "Doctor Lang and George Chapman". A victim of breast cancer, she had suffered a serious relapse in 1957, six months after a hospital operation. She was given a "no hope" verdict by a doctor who asked: "Surely you were aware you had cancer?" But Nurse Perry did not despair. A convinced Spiritualist—"I was born into it" she told me—she became one of the first patients to attend the Birmingham "house" clinic. Recalling that experience, she said that during the subsequent spirit "operation" she had clairvoyantly "seen" the entranced medium as "bearded". On her second visit, when she was introduced to

George Chapman prior to his going into trance, she had been surprised to find him clean-shaven and looking much younger than the man she had seen in trance.

As a result of inquiries through a friend she was sent a photograph of William Lang. "I recognized him immediately," she said. "It was the man I had 'seen' when the medium was entranced."

After six visits Mrs Perry was healed. Subsequent X-rays taken in a Manchester hospital baffled the doctors. She was told, "There is no trace of malignancy." At the time I met her this vital, laughing woman had herself become a healer. She believed that she and other members in her healing circle were often helped by Lang.

The clinic came into being as a result of another notable healing. Mrs Hilda Carter, of Woodville Road, Birmingham, acting-president of the Silver Street church which neighbours the "clinic", was healed by Lang of bowel trouble. She was cured during one of the healer's visits to a young crippled woman in her Birmingham home. Mrs Carter had sought earlier help from other healers, but without marked effect. Impressed in her friend's home by the speed and success of the Chapman-Lang ministration she asked him if he would be willing to come and treat other Birmingham friends who needed help. He agreed. Chapman treated twenty people in a group in a friend's home. The "clinic" was later opened in 1957 and Mrs Carter told me: "Through the years I have seen wonderful cures."

Mrs Beatrice Hilda Withers, who cheerfully presided over the improvised tea-and-sandwiches buffet on the day of my visit, also had a healing story to tell. She described Lang's 1962 spinal healing as "one of the most wonderful things that ever happened to me." At 8 a.m. on a Sunday morning she had fallen on ice-covered steps outside her home, fracturing her spine and cracking a hip bone. She was carried indoors and placed on a couch by her son. Mrs Withers had long been receiving beneficial healing through Chapman for an "incurable" discharging cyst, so she decided to put through a personal call to the medium's Aylesbury home. George came to the phone. Before the suffering woman had a chance to explain her plight, he said: "You've had a fall and hurt yourself, haven't you?" He told her he would go at once to his healing sanctuary to give absent healing, adding that she must also contact her own doctor.

Subsequently she was taken to the Silver Street clinic and given treatment. After she returned home she recalls: "I felt pain in my spine, and then suddenly felt my back go into position." When she visited a Birmingham hospital, two or three days later, to be told the results of nine X-rays which had previously been taken, one of the two hospital doctors present expressed astonishment that she was on her feet.

Showing her the plates which depicted crushed vertebrae, he expressed his bewilderment to his colleague. She was ordered back to bed, and instructed to return a week later by ambulance for a plaster corset. When the ambulance called with stretcher bearers she again astonished them by "being up and dressed". Friends still call her "the little miracle".

In this "spirit" clinic it was not only the complete absence of pills, drugs, disinfectants and surgical instruments which surprised! It was the pervading good will, astonishing stories and general expression of restored hope which impressed me. Patient after patient to whom I talked volunteered amazement, not only at Lang's accurate diagnoses, but at his knowledge and concern for unvoiced problems.

Miss Monica Norris, of Acocks Green, Birmingham, who told me she was "feeling much better mentally and physically" after only a second visit, added shyly: "It is such a pleasure to come here." Eagerly she was taken up by a nearby middle-aged housewife who had just emerged from the "surgery" after spirit treatment for fibroids. "What do you think the doctor greeted me with?" she asked. "He inquired, 'How's your daughter?' I told him, 'She's just had an operation.' He replied: 'I know, your husband's here. He told me'." She confessed to me that before leaving home, she had picked up a photograph of her "dead" husband and asked him to accompany her.

Similarly, Malcolm Smith, 32, proud owner of a three-wheeler car built for the disabled, who had driven down from Rotherham, in Yorkshire, also told me: "I'm so glad I've met Doctor Lang. He even answers your unspoken questions." Smith, who broke his spine three years earlier in a motor-cycle accident, said he had come to Silver Street as a last hope. After seeing the hospital X-rays an osteopath had told him he could not continue treatment. But when I talked to him Smith told me the excruciating muscular spasms in his legs had almost vanished as a result of the Chapman-Lang treatments. Smilingly he said he had recently "taken a six-mile walk over the moors" to test out the growing strength of his legs.

In recent years increasing pressure of work has forced George Chapman to give up his Birmingham clinic, but he continues to receive a monthly coach-load of thirty patients from Birmingham who travel to Aylesbury for necessary treatment.

But on that particular Saturday the Birmingham healing session lasted half an hour longer than the normal six hours, because there were so many new patients. Indeed in poignant circumstances, a blind eye was turned on the wall notice which read: "Mr Chapman regrets that patients without appointments will not be able to see Dr Lang."

The rule was broken when an obviously very sick 45-year-old man turned up unexpectedly. His actual appointment was not until February 12, but he said desperately, "I've felt so ill I had to come today."

He was quickly admitted into the healing sanctuary where I was privileged to help him on to the medical couch prior to an examination and subsequent spirit "operation" carried out with delicacy, speed and skill.

I learned that the man had been sent home from hospital where doctors had diagnosed an inoperable intestinal tumour. Accurately Lang described to the patient his hidden fears and physical symptoms of gnawing pain and repetitive nausea. No promises were given, but the treatment proposed by the "surgeon" was detailed to the patient in terms a layman could easily understand. Above all, reassurance was given and a degree of lost hope restored, perhaps because Lang conveyed that little extra—an atmosphere of loving concern—which can and *does* achieve marvels.

On another occasion a very happy man walked into my London newspaper office to tell me how he had been saved from incipient blindness by the "dead" surgeon working through the Aylesbury healer. My visitor was the Czech journalist and best-selling author of half-a-dozen books on espionage and politics, J. Bernard Hutton.

Later he not only dedicated his seventh brain product *Out of this World* to William Lang and George Chapman, "the wonderful spirit doctor and his medium who saved and greatly improved my once hopeless eyesight", but additionally wrote a psychic best-seller *Healing Hands* which provides a fascinating, copiously-documented biographical portrait of the Chapman-Lang partnership.

The story of that partnership is fascinating. George Chapman, born on February 4, 1921, in Merseyside's dockland, was brought up by grandparents. It was a tough setting for any sensitive youngster for in those between-the-wars years Merseyside was officially designated a "Depressed Area". But the grey-skied north and its warmhearted citizens bequeathed to George an invaluable heritage of guts, kindliness, abundant common-sense and humour.

When George left school he took a variety of hard-won jobs. They included those of garage hand, butcher and dock worker. Later he joined the R.A.F. and became an instructor in gunnery, boxing and battle drill. In 1943 he was transferred to Buckinghamshire where he met Margaret, the girl who was to become his devoted wife.

In *The Richest Vein*, an autobiographical booklet which I cherish, George has told part of his moving psychic experiences, which followed the death of the first child of that marriage. The baby, Vivian Margaret Chapman, survived less than one month. Movingly the healer writes: "I now believe, with all my heart, that God sent Vivian to us on a two-fold mission, to strengthen us spiritually and to draw us closer in the knowledge, love and fellowship of God. . . . It has been said that tragedy and sorrow never leave us where we were originally. We are grateful to God for the privilege of learning some great truths through His tiny messenger, Vivian Margaret Chapman."

When Spiritualists told him this child would grow up in another world, George decided to find out for himself whether there was "anything in it". "At first," he told me, "I was introduced into a development circle. The sitters were sincere but I felt I could develop better if I sat alone. I believed I was master of my own mind and that no harm could come to me. So I sat alone at home, using our bedroom. Marge helped me a great deal. She and I would discuss my progress.

"Whenever local Spiritualists invited a medium to take a group sitting I would attend. Mediums always advised me against sitting alone, but I felt I knew what I was doing. But I agree that normally a really well-run circle guided by a good medium is best. I would certainly never advise persons to sit alone unless they have this inner certainty and self-discipline."

Roy Morgan was one of the first mediums to tell Chapman he had a healing gift. Later other mediums confirmed this. They were proved correct. Chapman's heretical method of awakening his fine psychic powers proved amply justified by the end result.

One of the happenings which helped to convince George that he had the healing gift is told by Bernard Hutton in *Healing Hands*. In 1946, George, who had joined the Aylesbury Fire Brigade, was hurrying along to work when he saw an old man standing help-lessly on the kerb. George took his arm and helped him cross the busy road. Hutton tells us: "As he held the stranger's arm, Chapman realized that the old man could hardly have any use of the limb, so locked did it feel in its bent position. He made no comment, however, but laid his free hand on the fixed joint. When they reached the other side of the road the old man suddenly shouted: 'It's free. It's free!' Chapman did not say anything. He left the stranger and walked quickly away. When he had gone some little way, he looked back and saw the old man still standing on the edge of the pavement, moving his arm up and down and crying excitedly: 'He's made it move!'"

Hutton, in an astonishing chapter "The Moment of Death", also tells the story of a tape recording he made of a "trance" interview when Lang described his after-death experiences and how George Chapman had been found and trained to act as his earthly vehicle for trance "operations". Lang had related how after death "you retain the same personality as you had on earth". He had retained his passion to continue the art of medicine and told how he had been trained on the other side to acquire the "vastly different" techniques involved in the art of spirit surgery.

When he had finally asked if he could be allowed to help people suffering from serious ailments on earth he had been told that the only way this could be done was "to find a medium for you through whom you could reappear on the earth plane. It is very hard to find the *right* medium, but it is possible."

Eventually the medium was found, prepared and tested, and in his *Healing Hands* biography Hutton details 153 case-histories of interviewed patients who claimed to have been "cured completely and lastingly" as a result of this notable two worlds partnership. It should be noted, too, that Hutton has only included named patients who were also willing fully to substantiate their statements.

Lang also told Hutton: "No healer should ever discourage a

patient from attending a doctor—in fact he should always advise his patient to seek the help of the medical profession. Whenever possible, doctors should be told when their patients are receiving spirit healing. There should be the fullest co-operation between the two professions because each can learn much from the other."

Characteristically, Lang lost no time in trying to help George Chapman to secure not only full corroboration of the earthly identity of his "spirit control" but also eventual recognition from former patients, such as Mrs Bailey and from doctors who had worked with Lang on earth.

In 1958 when Chapman was in trance Lang dictated the following letter to the Registrar of Moorfields Eye Hospital.

"I know that this is a strange letter for your hospital to receive, but both I and my son Basil were active members of your staff for many years.

"If you will look into my past records you will find much about me, e.g. I wrote a book entitled *The Medical Examination of the Eye* and my son wrote a number of books on the examination of and approach to a patient.

"It is my wish to invite members of your active medical staff, or indeed past members, to contact my medium, George Chapman, with the view to having appointments with me.

"I know that in eye surgery and technique I can be of great help and I am sure that many of the staff who are so interested and love their work will enjoy meeting me."

No direct reply was ever received to his remarkable letter but over the years medical interest in the posthumous activities of William Lang has mounted in various ways and when the full story can be told of the two worlds healing partnership at Aylesbury it will substantiate to a remarkable degree that "Mr Lang's great hope of building a bridge of understanding between orthodox medicine and spirit healing" was not illusory.

Following later contacts with hospitals where William Lang had formerly worked George Chapman aroused the interest of some of the surgeon's earthly contemporaries. Subsequent strict cross-examination and investigation of trance statements made by Lang in the presence of a group of these doctors finally satisfied them that they were faced with a riddling phenomenon of undoubted validity.

George consented to further sustained investigations and I have his permission to state that for many years fruitful investigations have continued under a "gentleman's" agreement.

While professional privacy must be respected in regard to the fruits of this agreement it can be stated in these pages that the "dead" surgeon certainly succeeded in fully convincing at least one hard-headed London practitioner, who can be named. He was the late Dr Kildare Lawrence Singer of Hayes, Middlesex, whom William Lang had instructed in advanced ophthalmology techniques many years ago at Middlesex Hospital. The sequel to his first meeting with the posthumous Lang in the healing sanctuary at St Bride's, home of the Chapman family, has been described by my journalist colleague and friend, Roy Stemman, in an article published in *Psychic News* on May 22, 1965.

Dr Singer had become ill in the early '60s. The diagnosis was cancer, complicated by a heart disease which ruled out an operation. Finally he was persuaded to make an appointment to see Chapman's spirit collaborator, William Lang. As in the case of Mrs Bailey, recognition was mutual and immediate. Stemman wrote: "For Dr Singer it was a revelation. As well as the intimate details of life at the Middlesex, which only a person there at the time would have known, Dr Singer was also stunned by the wealth of medical knowledge of the homely old surgeon. 'He was shattered by the experience,' said Mrs Singer."

Dr Singer received healing during two visits. He was able to discard his formerly rigid invalid diet and his passing in 1961 was a result of a thrombosis. He had continued his work as a G.P. until the eve of his death.

Early the following year Dr Singer's widow and his daughter, Arlene Singer, at that time a ground hostess at London airport, received a surprise invitation to visit "Mr Lang" at Aylesbury. They did so and the spirit surgeon revealed that during his visits to see Lang, Dr Singer had asked him to try to "get hold of my daughter so that I can try to use her for healing after my own passing".

During that memorable afternoon Lang carried out a test which satisfied him that Arlene Singer could be used as a medium for healing. She agreed and for a year she regularly attended monthly healing sessions at Aylesbury where she was trained in the art of spirit healing, guided by her father.

During these training sessions Dr Singer made it known that he wished his old surgery to be converted into a sanctuary so that he could continue, through his daughter, his healing work in Hayes. His wish has been carried out and Lang predicted that eventually she would find it necessary to devote herself full time to healing the sick.

I can only say that I agree wholeheartedly with the view expressed by Bernard Hutton. Though neither George Chapman nor William Lang has ever claimed that the healing of any spectacular case has been the result of a miracle—miracles *do* happen at Aylesbury.

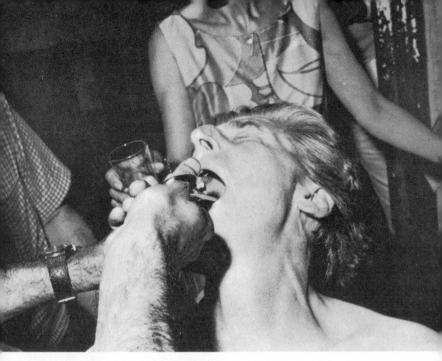

1. *Scissor insertion in mouth prior to removal of author's tonsils (Copyright: Hess)*

2. *The T-shaped scars, with blood flowing from the razor scar (Copyright: Hess)*

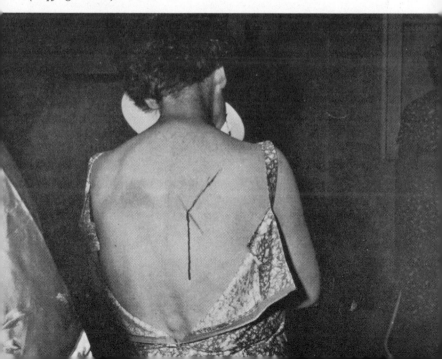

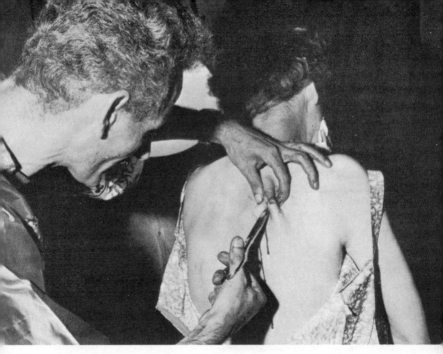

3. *De Freitas uses scissor points to open the scar (Copyright: Hess)*

4. *De Freitas sucks out a coagulated blood clot from the author's back (Copyright: Hess)*

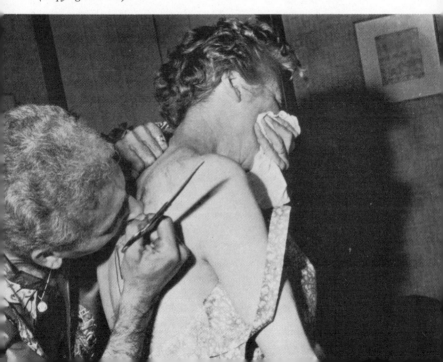

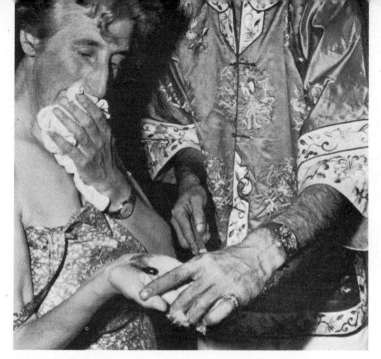

5. *The blood clot sucked from the back wound (Copyright: Hess)*

6. *The stitches are pulled up to encourage full blood flow (Copyright: Hess)*

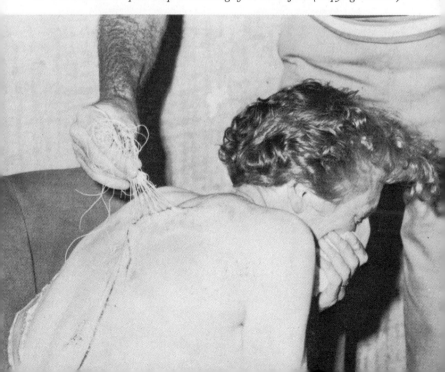

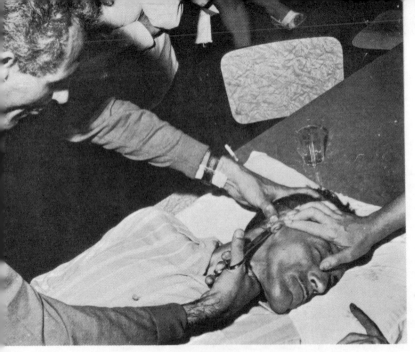

7. *A mastoid operation (Copyright: Hess)*

8. *De Freitas stitches the wound after the operation (Copyright: Hess)*

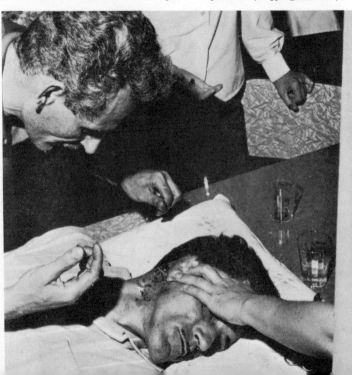

6. Lourival

June 10, 1966, is a date I'm never likely to forget, though it began normally enough, commuting to my London office at *Psychic News* in Great Queen Street. I had spent a pleasantly routine morning telephoning news contacts and carrying out background research in the newspaper's extensive files.

Thirty-five years of peripatetic reporting and roving wage-earning had expanded the waistline and silvered my hair. Worse, they had also substantially eroded youth's zestful confidence in life's limitless capacity to erupt into the sensational.

How mistaken I was! For Chance, Destiny, call it what you will, was already preparing a bombshell which was eventually to catapult me out of a cosy desk job across continents and oceans on a still unfinished fact-finding mission which to date has already logged over 11,000 miles by land, sea and air.

Its time fuse began to burn when an afternoon buzz from the internal telephone summoned me to the editor's office to "take off his hands" two strangers who had apparently arrived without prior warning.

Waving a hand in the direction of his visitors the editor, Maurice Barbanell, invited me "to meet one of Brazil's leading 'psychic surgeons'." Shaking hands with a handsome, grizzle-haired six-footer, Lourival de Freitas, I learned from his friend, who spoke excellent English, that they had just flown in from Rio de Janeiro.

As they returned with me to my office I hastily recalled fantastic tales I had read of untutored healer-mediums in Brazil and in the Philippines. They had been dubbed "psychic surgeons" because of their reputed, extraordinary ability to perform danger-ous surgical operations on medical incurables without any of the normal orthodox aids such as anaesthetics or sterilized medical equipment.

In the ensuing half-hour my initial interest deepened to a sense of stupefaction as I was shown colour photographs of extruded eyeballs and patients bleeding after kitchen knife extractions of apparent tumours while fully conscious.

The startling pictures recalled to my mind the strange tale told to me two years earlier by a former veteran colleague, Mrs Ethel Rosenthal. She had returned from a Brazilian cruise, haunted and disturbed by her own eyewitness experience of operations similar to those depicted in the photographs I was holding in my hands.

They had been performed, she said, by a Brazilian taxi-driver whom she only knew as "Mr X" because the operations he carried out were illegal in Brazil, even though "X" never accepted any payment for them.

She related how this man, using an unsterilized kitchen knife, had thrust it under a girl's eyelid, and then laid a growth on her cheek. The girl had appeared to feel no pain and had later danced and drank with other guests present.

As I told this to my visitors they exchanged quizzical glances and began to smile. The penny dropped! Mr "X" and Lourival de Freitas were one and the same person, but he had changed his job in the interim period.

Sensing my intense interest I was invited to accompany them that evening to witness a private demonstration of Lourival's healing skill, on the understanding that I attended in a personal capacity and not as a professional journalist primarily seeking a story. I gladly accepted.

After dining in a West End restaurant we were taken by car to an attractive, middle-class home in Wimbledon. That evening, towards midnight, in the presence of seven other adult witnesses, I watched what I can only describe as the medically unbelievable and the scientifically impossible.

During conversation at dinner I had already been informed that Lourival never claimed any personal credit for any successes which might result from his healing ministrations. He regarded himself, I was told, "as merely a channel for God's work carried out by the team of 'spirit' healers and doctors who use his body while he is in trance."

Trance is a mysterious and frequently encountered psychic phenomenon. Little is scientifically known about its true nature although its varying physiological characteristics are well-known. These can range from a state of apparent sleep, or suspended consciousness, to an extreme of cataleptic rigidity. Usually a deep-trance medium brings back little or no remembrance of what has passed in the trance and personality changes can be striking.

As I first discovered on that memorable night of June 10, Lourival's form of trance represents a state of complete withdrawal of his normal consciousness, a withdrawal he appears to achieve with effortless ease and rapidity after bending forward, head dropped. Simultaneously his breathing undergoes a marked change, outwardly characterized by an audible gasp. When he quickly straightens up again an extraordinary change in personality is immediately apparent. It is so complete that it has been described by one expert observer, himself a deep trance medium, as "possession". Certainly, in Lourival's case, this change is accompanied not only by increased physical vigour but also by a markedly enhanced psychological, emotional and mental range.

On June 10 he was successively controlled by two contrasting personalized forces—the first a male claiming to be Nero, the Roman Emperor of ill-repute, the second a woman said to be a member of Nero's entourage. Psychiatrists, of course, would dismiss these "spirit controls" as merely "secondary personalities" created in the medium's subconscious. Whatever the true explanation, their advent on June 10 produced remarkable personality switches in the entranced man.

During a 3½-hour trance, undisturbed by a thunderstorm of dramatic intensity, Lourival smoked at intervals between operations and drank copious draughts of undiluted whisky as an aid to deepen trance or to induce change of "spirit" control. Yet, when he is not in a trance state the medium is a strict teetotaller. I can personally attest that in subsequent months when I saw much of him the only out-of-trance occasion on which I saw him persuaded to drink a glass of wine produced an unfortunate result. He became violently sick.

An English doctor who accompanied me some weeks later to another, and more controversial, demonstration of Lourival's psychic powers, during which the entranced healer had gulped down the contents of a large bottle of whisky in one go, described the feat as "supernormal". Commenting on the strange fact that Lourival remained physically unaffected—even his breath bore no trace of alcohol—the doctor told me that if a normal man had drunk even two-thirds of that amount of alcohol at similar speed, he would have endangered his life and would certainly have fallen into a prolonged alcoholic coma.

The peak moment for me on that unforgettable June evening came when, standing close to the medium under the bright light of a central chandelier in the living room of my English hosts, I watched him "operate" upon the back of their delicate, six-year-old daughter, protectively held by her mother.

Having pressed the cotton-wool protected rim of a large crystal tumbler on the child's back Lourival slowly revolved the glass. In the course of doing so he also asked the child's grandfather to place his hand on the tumbler which Lourival continued to guide. Sensing the unavoidable tension of the watching adults, the child began to whimper. The whimper rose to a momentary wail as I watched in stupefaction the slow-motion emergence of what I later described as a "sculptured rose" of evilly discoloured tissue which *grew* to thumbnail size before dropping off the child's back into the enclosing glass. The child's flesh through which it had so unaccountably processed bore no scar. For the rest of the evening, submerged in surgical spirit, the fleshy "rose" in the tumbler remained the sole tell-tale witness of the incredible "operation".

The little girl, triumphantly carried off to her waiting nursery cot, bore neither scar nor bruise to testify to the night's experience. For her it was the end of years of suffering and illness. I learned that from the age of eighteen months she had suffered from an acute bronchial condition, later diagnosed as bronchiectasis, which involves the secretion of mucus in the lung. Underweight, thin and pale, she had also had pneumonia. A patch on one lung and a heart murmur had also been medically detected. In the care of a chest consultant she was given continuous anti-biotic treatment, coupled with daily postural drainage at home. But her general condition worsened and the parents had been warned that if there was no improvement a lobectomy, an operation entailing removal of the lower right-hand lobe of her lung, could ultimately be necessary. Meanwhile the parents had been advised to give their daughter the benefit of sea air. They planned to move to the South coast.

On that same evening, a second, unscheduled, "spirit" operation took place when I had left the room for a brief period. It was performed on the back of the neck of the child's father. When I returned my companions drew my attention to a second tumbler containing blood-stained cerebral tissue. They informed me that after making a surface scratch on the patient's neck with a needle, the medium had then sucked out the diseased matter into his own mouth, later rinsed out with surgical spirit.

When I had re-entered the room I found the patient stretched out in an apparent faint on a couch. Later he confirmed that he had been unconscious of what had happened. Fully revived he gaily questioned those who had been present about what had taken place. He told me : "I experienced no pain and remember nothing except that I appeared to be holding a conversation with my subconscious; I cannot recall what it was about."

Lourival, who is skilled in herbal lore, also gave his adult patient strips of a resinous bark brought from Brazil. He was instructed to break this into small pieces and to steep each section overnight in a tumbler containing water. The infusion was to be drunk daily on awakening. He also gave his host spirit-dictated advice concerning recommended future action.

The enormous energy expenditure required by the Brazilian's unusual trance-healing techniques was strikingly illustrated in the final treatment carried out that evening.

In this instance the patient was a sceptical linguistics professor, said to be a victim of insomnia and nervous tension which doctors had been unable to alleviate to any appreciable extent. Lourival, still in trance, had commenced his treatment by making darting lightning-speed passes with his hands around the patient's body. The professor, who appeared to have fallen unconscious from his chair to the floor, was then flung over the healer's shoulder and shaken vigorously, head downwards, as if he had been a sack of potatoes. Still unconscious, the man was then placed on the couch. After further passes his skull was tapped with a long-handled brass spoon. Treatment ended with a request from Lourival that we should all stand up, encircling the patient with linked hands. A prayer was then recited.

Later, the professor, revived and very cheerful, told me : "I remember nothing of the healing treatment except for the brief moment when I smelled the carpet." He was alluding to his fantastic, fish-like leap from his chair, face downward on the carpet, when he himself apparently became entranced by the healer's "passes".

The postscript to that landmark evening of June 10, came nine months later after my return from Brazil, when I visited the new seaside home of the child patient. Her high spirits, good appetite and freedom from her former chronic cough were eloquent proofs of restored vitality.

Here is her happy father's own account of his child's astonishing cure :

Our daughter made an immediate, dramatic and instantaneous recovery. On the very next day she raided the fridge and would not stop eating; this was totally unlike her previous attitude towards food. Her cheeks had better colour and she was noticeably more relaxed and cheerful. From that day to this she just hasn't looked back. She has not even caught a common cold when the rest of us have had colds, whereas previously she had been the first to catch anything going. We then moved down here. A subsequent medical examination showed that her lungs were now clear, there was no more blockage of congealed phlegm and her heart murmur has also gone. She was declared fit. It may well be that our daughter had something even more serious wrong with her; the doctors were not very forthcoming.

Try and put yourself in our shoes as the parents : there were not just a few weeks of anxiety over her health, but *years*. It was with us all the time. Then, suddenly, it went. Bronchiectasis *on its own* may be subject to spontaneous recovery, but not when it is accompanied by other complications and has reached the stage of a proposed lobectomy. Besides, even spontaneous recovery does not usually mean *overnight* recovery with something like bronchiectasis. If it gets better on its own it improves gradually, not with such dramatic suddenness.

He also commented :

On such occasions doctors like to say that the initial diagnosis must have been mistaken. Personally I do not believe that such a cure can be explained in terms of mere coincidence or auto-suggestion. So far as my wife and I are concerned, a Brazilian medium who would be classified by many as a primitive witch doctor has cured our daughter of a condition which orthodox medicine had been unable to deal with.

We are also impressed by the fact that de Freitas has since refused absolutely to accept any form of payment, or even a token of our profound gratitude. His view is that whatever healing forces operate through him are at the free disposal of his fellow-men.

I have since learned that his view is shared by all genuine Brazilian mediums.

In a later article published in the *London Hospital Gazette* (vol. lxxl, March 1968, pp. 17–18) the father described the "glass operation" and explained the circumstances which had led to it. He wrote :

My wife is Brazilian, and her uncle knew the medium well and had seen several of his "psychic operations". When he visited this country it was suggested that he might be able to help our daughter's condition, and as we were so anxious about her long-term health, we were willing to try anything and agreed to invite the medium to our home. My wife and I had no experience of psychic phenomena but had implicit faith in the judgement and sound sense of my wife's uncle, who is down-to-earth and a prominent executive in Brazil. He assured us that no harm would come to our child and his assurances are meaningful. We were understandably sceptical but after seeing what we did, have no doubt that this phenomenon was real. This does not mean that we accept all psychic phenomena on hearsay : we only accept this because it was part of our own experience.

This case must obviously strain credulity for those raised in the standard medical tradition, but more things exist than are in medical textbooks and it would be a dull world if there were not. It is a mistake to dismiss all "fringe medicine" as superstition and quackery or both, when cures *do* take place. The proper reaction to any cure is surely to rejoice rather than just to criticize, so one should first investigate for oneself. If doctors are not prepared to do this then they should not judge.

In his concluding passage he urged doctors to be open-minded.

He wrote : "It is too easy to dismiss all this as 'primitive sorcery' or 'voodoo', although these phenomena are all too often linked with undesirable association; but these are probably necessary for primitive people and we should not be put off by them. I believe that there is now substantial evidence to support this remarkable phenomenon, which deserves further investigation. Surely one must examine the evidence and witness their work before pronouncing."

7. Under the Knife

How does it feel to be a guinea-pig for psychic surgery? It's not an easy question to answer. Certainly it bequeathes a permanent fellow sympathy with guinea-pigs in general and those of science in particular.

Then, of course, there is also the tricky problem of trying, with what honesty you can muster, to assess just where you yourself stand within this experimental hierarchy. That's one probably only the guinea-pig could answer and most likely it wouldn't be flattering to any human ego. One thing's for sure, I'm a cowardly field specimen.

Before my own 35-minute ordeal it was touch and go whether I stayed or fled. Fortunately, circumstances took a ruthless jump forward before I'd finally opted for the irremediable. For that I'm glad . . . very!

This is not a story about any claimed "miracle" cure, for my heretical medical adventure led to medical controversy, not only about the nature of the methods used but also the degree of improvement.

Nevertheless, I shall always be grateful to Lourival who, rejecting payment, unhesitatingly risked his own freedom to carry out an "illegal" operation on a patient medically classified over twenty years earlier as suffering from bronchiectasis.

Victim of a half-pint lung haemorrhage, following a dental operation under an anaesthetic in February, 1946, I had been admitted as an emergency patient to St Bartholomew's hospital, Smithfield, London.

The subsequent fourteen days' investigations provided ample opportunity for doleful bed ponderings on whether the verdict would turn out to be tuberculosis or lung abscess. The former was a probability so strongly favoured by my own worried G.P. that she had lost no time in notifying the local authority of the need to disinfect my flat. On the other hand, lung abscess was the No 1 "suspect" of the hospital outpatients' doctor, who, after examination, brusquely forbade me to walk any further in the direction of home than the nearest vacant bed in an upstairs ward.

Neither proved good tipsters. Eventually told by a solemn young "intern" that I was suffering from an inoperable lung condition arising from a too-long standing dilation of the bronchi, I smiled and remarked, "Well, *that's* a relief." Having survived a childhood dominated by the dismal insignia of countless cartons of cough mixtures and seemingly bottomless jars of malodorous cod liver oil, bronchiectasis for me merely represented a *named* extension of all too familiar discomforts.

Rejoicing at the prospect of home and liberty I listened with euphoric detachment to a medical lecture on the perils of my condition, the folly of smoking, and the need, twice daily for the rest of my life, to carry out postural drainage. In layman's language this means hanging upside down like a bat for as long as you can bear the ludicrous indignity and resulting blinding headache. He also warned: "Take life slowly since you must realize you only have three-fifths of the normal lung capacity."

Thus firmly placed on the medical shelf at 34, I made three or four serious attempts to give up smoking, but on each occasion found the resulting irritability, depression and general nervousness caused by the virtue of abstinence harder to bear than the physical price to be paid for continued addiction to the infernal weed.

Not surprisingly, the "inoperable" verdict was re-confirmed in 1959 by a Sussex chest specialist. He told me that my ability to remain in any full-time professional employment must become increasingly dependent upon regular supplies of costly, health-service supplied antibiotics to help ward off acute bronchial attacks and their inevitable concomitant haemoptysis. The latter tongue-twister is merely a medical euphemism for blood-spitting.

Unorthodox preparations for the operation began in an unexpected way. During a Sunday car trip to a beautiful tropic waterfall Lourival waded into the river and plucked a large sharp-edged reed. Using this as an improvized razor-blade, he proceeded to notch an oblique scar under my right shoulder blade. After examination he pronounced with satisfaction that "the way the cut had taken" ensured it would be possible to carry out the projected glass-cupping operation six days later to bring about a hoped-for 40 to 70 per cent improvement in my present condition.

In the intervening days herbal treatment was given. I was ordered to drink four wineglassfuls daily of a pleasant tasting syrupy lemon-mint mixture prepared by the healer. It certainly proved effective in lessening my normally profuse bronchial catarrh. Additionally, I was instructed to drink several tumblers daily of a nauseous tasting brownish herbal tea, a remedy said to clear excess liquid from the kidneys.

Told it would be harmful to continue excessive smoking during the treatment I rashly agreed to cut it out altogether. This abrupt cessation of my normal 30–35 cigarette intake undoubtedly contributed to resulting bouts of depression, particularly immediately prior to the "operation". Subconscious fear was probably a subsidiary cause. My self-imposed ban, by the way, lasted a mere sixty days.

In the session about to be described the healer worked in the harsh light of unshaded electric bulbs and an additional portable standard lamp for maximum light when actually operating. Spectators and patients present varied from a dozen to fifteen throughout the evening. Lourival himself never left the operating arena which consisted of two large adjoining rooms linked by a wide arch.

Before I give my own necessarily subjective impressions here is an eyewitness account written for me by a Brazilian friend present on that evening. He is a man who had considerable prior knowledge of psychic surgery procedures and he accepts their validity.

JOURNALIST'S EYEWITNESS REPORT

"Nero", Lourival's chief spirit control, "came down" at about ten o'clock and held up proceedings for the arrival of a further three invited guests. The delay seemed to make Nero irritable but when the expected guests arrived the session opened with an eye operation on an elderly man. This man had previously been successfully operated on by the medium for a leg infection which doctors had failed to heal. In full light the medium inserted a knife under the man's eyelid, then with a pair of scissors cut and brought out a cheese-like substance, stating this had been causing an infection which was retarding the complete healing of the leg. The patient was very quiet and calm throughout the eye operation and, indeed, was soon afterwards joining in the singing.

Fifteen minutes later "Nero" was on the verge of his second operation, with agitation building up in the form of a tirade against the press, creating a very tense uncomfortable atmosphere.*

It was explained to us later that "Nero" was not in command, but rather Lourival's Japanese control, Sheka. The latter is said to be the only one of the medium's spirit guides who has expertise in the kind of bronchus and lung operation which they intended to do on Anne that evening.

The second operation was performed on J.'s baby daughter, and proved to be a glandular operation. She seemed to be frightened and cried out but as soon as it was over she became peaceful and was placed in a big armchair in the rear recess to rest. She soon seemed to sleep quietly.

Next we knew the child's mother was lying on the sofa. With a glass which a nearby woman helper was asked to press down deeply into the patient's flesh "Nero" removed what he later said was a stomach ulcer, though the glass was held in the womb area and what came out seemed much bigger than an ulcer. The medium then stepped on the patient's stomach. She seemed to feel nothing at all.

There followed an interval during which "Nero's" verbal tirade grew in violence. Indeed he seemed to be nervous and irritable with everybody except P. whom he kept on praising. Within the half hour a third operation comprised the removal of what was termed a skin wart from the woman helper who had been asked to press down the glass for the "ulcer" operation. This was quickly over.

Then followed another tense interval, during which "Nero" picked on an interview Anne had undertaken that day with a

* Tension can sometimes be marked in varying forms of physical phenomena. Some researchers believe it performs a useful purpose to "strike" or draw psychic power from individuals in the audience. Certainly it is an effective method of establishing quick domination over an audience. A.D.

former patient, suggesting this action had had a damaging effect. This was more pretext than fact, since I myself had been present. I became concerned as to whether the projected "operation" on Anne should continue but avoided approaching her lest this should be the excuse for further outbursts. However, she somehow stood the tide and later, standing up in the room, she was asked to open her mouth to enable her throat to be examined.

She was told her tonsils would have to be removed. There was some difficulty in controlling her tongue. Finally, with the back of the handle of a spoon the medium managed to hold it down. He then plunged his scissors into her throat, hacking away for about two minutes. Anne seemed to be releasing some of her pent-up nervousness in the form of a feeling of pain. She was obviously distressed. However, she did not cry out as she thought she did, but no doubt "inside her" she was. Certainly the operation was more brutal than any I have hitherto seen in a "psychic" throat operation.

"Nero" operated with his mouth open in a circle, whereas he usually has his tongue between his lips. Obviously Sheka was in command but there must have been some hitch in the union between the spiritual entity and Lourival's physical body. Nonetheless the operation continued to its conclusion when darkish matter was extracted—about the size of a baby's fist.

Later "Nero" explained the operation had included not only the tonsils but also a complete cleaning out of the bronchi. A spectator later commented, "He brought up everything but the kitchen sink."

Anyhow, Anne was allowed to take a few minutes' breather on a chair while further photographs were taken. Then she was asked to stand up again, her exposed back to the medium. He proceeded to cut the skin in the area where, on the previous Sunday, he had scarred it with the blade of a reed plucked from a mountain river. He then manipulated the skin, squeezing it and forcing it to bleed, to open the cut more widely.

When he had completed whatever he had to do he applied his mouth to the wound and started sucking with tremendous force. He then threw back his head, blood trickling over his lips to his chin. He slowly opened his mouth and from the tip of his tongue passed on to the palm of his hand a clot of black blood about half an inch long. He later said this had come from the patient's lung and in it was collected bacteria which was the cause of almost all the trouble. He did not rinse out his mouth immediately but later went into the rear recess. When he came back his mouth had no signs of blood. He had probably washed it out with alcohol. The final stitching took place while Anne lay face downwards on the couch which an earlier patient had been asked to vacate. It was noticeable that once the operation was over the medium became much calmer.

AUTHOR'S ACCOUNT

Having been told that the "surgery" session, due to commence at 8 p.m., would be devoted solely to my bronchus operation, I was surprised to find a number of unanticipated guests, most of them former patients or friends of Lourival.

In his first operation on the old man "Nero" removed a growth from the patient's right eye. This was photographed. Earlier a photograph was also taken of the man's almost healed leg. I myself was startled and impressed to note that within a fortnight the former gaping cavity had healed over with a light covering of new flesh.

During the second "op" of the evening, a glandular operation necessitated a neck incision. The child cried out piteously, but only during the actual cutting and speedy sucking out of tissue. I turned away and walked out of the open door because moment-arily I couldn't bear the child's apparent suffering. I had also earlier learned, in a hurried aside from "X", that "Nero" didn't want me to look at any operation. I imagine that my mounting nervousness was known and what was in store for me, too, though I myself was still banking on the promised "glass cupping" operation.

During "Nero's" ensuing long, angry tirade, which, I gathered from occasional words recognized here and there, included criticism of myself, I became increasingly depressed and tense. I again walked out of the room and stood in dejected indecision at the top of a flight of stone stairs leading to the garden below. I wanted to go right away but realized I couldn't commit the insult of a cowardly flight. I was doubly committed: personally I had gratefully agreed to the proposed imminent operation; profession-ally I had an unfinished duty on my hands for had I not travelled thousands of miles to study a man who, in my view, had unjustly been accused in England of trickery? And perhaps most important of all, here was a man bravely risking his own freedom to give unrecompensed help where it was badly needed, for on the day of our first meeting in England I had been sent from work to a London hospital for X-rays to ascertain the cause of renewed lung bleeding.

To ease my inward conflict I re-entered the room and went into the rear recess for a drink of water. Crossing to the open windows I looked out at the serene stars and tried to regain the rags of a restored courage, and composure. It was here that I myself was "caught" by the entranced Lourival.

The attitude of Lourival's "control", whom I still thought to be "Nero", was brutally brusque. The ensuing operation inside my throat was also unexpected and much grimmer than I had anticipated. I found it difficult to breathe when the large scissors began digging into my back palate, particularly as I was simultaneously being semi-dragged across the room to enable the medium to get better light. I was conscious of pain and fright, so much that I ashamedly thought I was screaming, though "X" assured me later I only grunted. I remember grasping P.'s arm to steady myself, for I was in doubt as to just how much longer I could keep on my feet and continue breathing. Then I heard P. say, "Relax, Anne, relax."

Then I found myself being handed a tumbler by P. and being told: "Don't cough. Just spit with all your might." I was photographed holding the tumbler now containing some mighty nasty stuff indeed. It seemed to be about a quarter full of tissue and a bloodied mixture. I was still spitting blood-stained mucus but was so relieved to be able to breathe freely once again I even found myself involuntarily laughing when someone jokingly called out, "Smile, Anne."

The second part of the operation began when I was asked to stand up again and I felt a razor blade lightly cutting into my flesh at right angles to the earlier reed scar. Then I could feel the medium's teeth grip and squeeze my flesh and I worried inwardly over how long I would be able to bear this if the pressure got much worse. But it was quickly over. I thought I had cried out again, but the pain wasn't nearly as bad as the throat operation had been. Next I found myself being handed a large clot of what looked like coagulated "black" blood about the size of an elongated coin but much thicker. I was very surprised at its blackness and shape.

The subsequent "stitching" as I lay face down on the couch—between nine and twelve individual stitches according to my rather confused counting—was unpleasant each time a fresh sewing needle plunged through the lips of the back cut. A good-hearted American friend standing nearby extended his hand, to which I clung. This gave me courage. Yet incredibly, those stitches were cut after about an hour. I felt very little pain and there was no bleeding. The sizeable scar site was then latticed over with strip bandaging by a gentle-fingered male helper.

Surprisingly, I never felt any further pain or the slightest discomfort from the scar on the upper part of my back but I had a bad 36 hours with my throat. Soon after the operation I began to spit up tiny pieces of torn flesh where the scissors had apparently dug into the palette. Was this due to the tonsils operation or had the "dematerialization" process of some of the ejected tissue been incomplete? I found it excruciating to swallow but Lourival proved to be a devoted "doctor". Within 24 hours, after being given salt gargles and an antibiotic tablet, I was drinking my first welcome cup of tea. Healing tissue was already forming over the throat lesions. But I got roundly scolded the morning after the operation when Lourival discovered that unaided I had pushed my rather heavy mahogany bed over to the window. Since I felt no discomfort whatever from the scar on my back I hadn't realized I was still running a very grave risk of re-opening the stitches under conditions where, so Lourival told me, it might have been impossible to staunch resultant bleeding.

I was instructed to take things very easy for ten days, during which time I was given eight Vitamin B injections, coupled with a course of calcium tablets. I felt well and the depth of my breathing—formerly increasingly shallow—was substantially increased. I no longer woke up feeling—as I had done for years prior to the operation—as if I was breathing over the top of a wall.

Within a week of my guinea-pig experience I wrote in a letter: "The medical efficacy of the operation will not be known until circumstances allow a full medical investigation to be carried out, if this eventually proves possible. But although my own experience was exceptional because I felt pain, I am so glad I went through with it. Irrespective of any X-ray results I can at least personally testify to my present substantial improvement—it is such a joy to be able to breathe deeply without obstruction. I can also personally testify that the tissue ejected orally and the blood clot taken from my back was not surreptitiously smuggled in from any butcher's shop as prejudiced English critics appear to have believed. The scar and more than thirty photographs taken also provide conclusive visual evidence that the experience was neither hypnotic nor merely hallucinatory."

8. Two Doctor Guinea-Pigs

"My medical colleagues can say what they like. Personally I have no doubt about the validity of the phenomenon. I can't explain how it originates. I only know that the psychic surgery operations I have seen carried out by my friend, Lourival de Freitas, are the most remarkable I have witnessed in my entire professional life."

The speaker, a man I had journeyed fourteen days across the Atlantic Ocean to interview in a colonial hill town in Brazil, was a stockily built, bright-eyed doctor in early middle age. His frank smile and easy gestures revealed a man on good terms with life. Similarly, his elegantly dressed artist wife, chattering toddler son, attractive home, well-kept lawns and English flower beds expressively indicated a happy domesticity and local success in his chosen field of medicine.

The doctor's collection of clocks softly intoned the passage of time, and the profiles of volcanic mountains gauntly sharpened in the deepening dusk of a December evening as he continued to enlarge upon two contrasted subjects each close to his heart—psychic surgery and poetry.

"When Lourival operates and cuts I have no doubt about it," he told me. "Using kitchen knives and scissors, without antiseptics or anaesthetics I have seen him painlessly extract stomach ulcers and tonsils, and carry out intestinal and womb operations. When Lourival put his knife into me for an intestinal operation I didn't feel anything, either during the cutting or during the subsequent stitching. The scar healed within twenty-four hours. I was astonished. True, the trouble wasn't completely healed up in my own case. Like every doctor Lourival can sometimes achieve a complete cure, sometimes only partial. He has his failures and I have also known some feel pain."

Apologizing—charmingly and unnecessarily—that he must ask me not to publish his name in regard to his testimony about "psychic surgery" which remains illegal under Brazilian law, my informant explained: "You will realize that my position is difficult professionally because many doctors don't share my views. During the period when I assisted as a friendly observer present during Lourival's psychic operations I met with considerable opposition and suspicion. But I am not naive. I know what I have seen and can confirm. You will also appreciate that when a doctor submits himself to an unorthodox operation as I have done it needs courage and faith especially because, professionally, you know so much about what is involved. Even the well-established fact that some psychic surgeons drink substantial quantities of alcohol while operating in trance violates biological laws. Yet in a single evening I have seen Lourival successively gulp down whisky, ether, champagne and cachaça" (a popular Brazilian spirit distilled from sugar cane).

When I asked him whether he thought psychic surgery a suitable subject for international study by doctors he replied without hesitation: "Yes, I would support this because there are things which my profession cannot solve. In the present stage of medical knowledge our only hope of solving them seems to lie in seeking spiritual help. Many illnesses cannot be treated with available medicines and, personally, I think it doubtful whether science will ever triumph unaided. That is why so many people, when they have lost all hope of earthly aid, turn to spiritual help —including psychic surgery, despite the present legal ban. Then again, why does a so-called "miracle" work with one person and not with another? I don't know but I do believe they *can* happen with spiritual help."

The doctor confessed that occasionally when he himself has been examining a patient he has become conscious of what he described as "spirit" help. "When I have placed my hands on the patient's head my eyes sometimes want to close and I have a hell of a job to keep them open. It is a sort of drowsiness but I fight it off because I want to carry out my medical diagnoses in my own way."

As we continued to chat over coffee the doctor's wife told me of her own successful sinus operation carried out some years earlier by Lourival. "Since then," she said, "I have prayed nightly in gratitude to his spirit guides who brought me such relief."

Recalling bygone years when Lourival had lived in the district, and been a frequent, welcome visitor to their home, she told me : "His services were so much in demand that he exhausted himself. Whenever he was here word mysteriously got around and patients would begin to turn up in their cars. These three rooms would be packed to overflowing and you would find more people anxiously waiting outside, not only in our garden but out in the road. But Lourival never accepted a penny for the operations he carried out."

Both the doctor and his wife confirmed the truth of a local event about which I was to hear much in my subsequent local enquiries concerning the efficacy of Lourival's "surgery". As the fame of his "illegal" cures had spread regional police had been ordered to investigate. Walking into a crowded late night session the detective had been spotted by the entranced medium who brusquely beckoned him over and told him, "You are ill." A successful operation was then performed upon the astonished man. Later, when this same detective was instructed to carry out the arrest of the medium, he told his chief : "You can send someone else. He cured me. I'm on his side."

And before I left the doctor told me a strange story of how he had witnessed a local firewalking session organized by Lourival. A local drunk who had sceptically watched some of his friends walk unharmed over the bed of glowing charcoal had boasted : "I don't believe in this stuff. Anyone can do it." Ignoring the medium's stern warning "not to try anything on his own, or he could not be responsible for the consequences", the tipsy man attempted to cross over the forbidden zone. He was taken to hospital, badly burned.

Walking through the quiet streets of the rural town back to my green-bowered, chalet hotel built on the lower slopes of a forest of eucalyptus trees, I was preoccupied by the many mysteries touched upon in our conversation. And I found myself wondering whether the doctor's parting prophecy might one day come true. He had told me : "You will find practically no atheists in Brazil. One day it will become a global centre for Spiritualism and occult knowledge because we not only enjoy racial tolerance but we are also a psychic people."

* * *

"Psychic surgery? Of course it is a reality! I've been a guinea-pig myself, for a septic appendix. And I don't mind confessing that knowing what was involved medically I had the wind up; yet I felt no pain and after three days there was not even a trace of the scar."

My smiling host who spoke with such frankness is a busy Rio doctor with specialist knowledge in tropical medicine. A man who makes no secret of his Spiritualist convictions he enjoys considerable repute both as a scientific researcher into the paranormal and as a witty erudite lecturer on the subject.

His enthusiastic audiences include student-priests and nuns.

Few men alive can equal his knowledge of the fantastic "art" of psychic surgery. Dr Cavalcanti Bandeira's four years' investigation of one of the Brazilian practitioners personally known to him was the subject of a striking, illustrated article, "Milagres de Barbosa" published in a Brazilian journal *Fatos e Fotos* (March 1966).

Telling me about the work of this extraordinary medium, as we turned the pages of extensive research files, Dr Bandeira said Barbosa had possessed an astonishing ability to "open up a body without instruments". Lightly passing a fingernail over the surface of cotton wool wadding placed over the site of the "operation", the medium would cause the flesh of the patient to open and "blood would soak up through the swab". Then, inserting scissors points, he brought out the diseased tissue. He would then close the wound by a mere movement of his fingers and apply a sticky plaster as a light bandage. When removed, three days later, there would be no trace of a scar.

Senhora Bandeira, like her husband, is a remarkable example of successful psychic surgery carried out by Lourival de Freitas. A woman of glowing vitality, she shares her husband's respect for the "miracles" of psychic surgery, exemplified in her own case by a successful major operation.

As she served refreshments in her lofty, colonial period drawing room, rich in medieval religious art, antique silver and crystal, a family friend present, a young naval surgeon, Dr Vilde, shyly summed-up for me what he described as the modern doctor's dilemma.

"Surgery," he said, "is becoming increasingly complex. Our trouble is that while we increasingly know the 'how' of a particular disease, we are little nearer knowing the whys and wherefores.

Why, for instance, does one man suddenly fall victim to a duodenal ulcer while another, who from the medical point of view would appear to be a much more likely subject, goes scot-free?"

Sharing his friends' enthusiasm for the paranormal, he told me of his own researches with a bearded, doctor-medium famed in Rio for what I can only term "instant" psycho-analysis. With the help of his Brahmin "control" the doctor-medium's on-the-spot diagnoses are said to have resulted in astonishing recoveries, not only from psychosomatic illnesses but also medically-resistant chronic diseases.

In one case witnessed by the surgeon, a stranger stricken with leg paralysis had been able to dispense with his sticks after the clairvoyant doctor-medium had bluntly told the patient that his long-standing hatred of his mother had caused the crippling disability. Telling the astonished man, "Now you must forgive her," the doctor-seer described how the man's mother had tried to poison him in childhood after he had unwittingly discovered her in the act of adultery.

Describing mediumship as a "super-normal phenomenon which does not depend either on morals or an individual's beliefs", Bandeira told me that in his view: "Thought is a form of energy which it has been amply proved can be transmitted via telepathy. Similarly in the form of object-reading, commonly known as psychometry, we witness the ability of thought to impregnate matter. This is the principle which underlines popular belief in the efficacy of the religious amulet or 'blessed' object."

Many doctors in Brazil, he said, were interested in psychic phenomena. In contrast to the pragmatic Behaviourist attitudes favoured by so many European and American doctors, he and other Brazilian colleagues tended towards an instinctive acceptance of spontaneous psychic phenomena, which they might be said to have imbibed with their mothers' milk. "We know very well," he said, "that you can't disclose man's spirit in a test tube, or define the range of a human mind on an encephalograph."

One of his dreams is to set up a study group centre for doctor-mediums. Bandeira himself is a gifted psychic, but as he sadly says: "Research costs plenty, especially since in Brazil we like to keep to our tradition that no honest medium can take a penny for his work."

This lithe, lively intellectual, who in the two years before I met him had cheerfully expended over two million cruzeiros (£350) of his wife's hard-earned money on assiduous psychic researches, and bringing people from distant states in Brazil, is a notable example of the ideals which have inspired Brazilian Spiritualism over the past century. He is also characteristic of many gifted doctors in Brazil who have been fascinated by the subject. It is not without significance, for example, that one of the most distinguished pioneering Spiritist groups in Brazil, named the "Group Confucius" after the name of the spirit doctor who "prescribed" through a member of the group (a Dr Siqueira Dias), was largely composed of homeopathic practitioners. This group, indeed, was the first to establish a free service of homeopathic medicines "prescribed" by their healing-mediums. This social service to the needy did much to set the seal on the charitable work which to this day remains the driving force behind Spiritism throughout this sub-continent.

Bandeira described Brazil as a vast laboratory of the spiritual and the psychic. "Here," he told me, "we do not look upon Spiritualism—or Spiritism as we call it—as a separate religion. For us, survival and spirit communication explain the basis of *all* religion. It is for this reason that the Catholic Church must be tolerant in Brazil. It has no choice in the matter."

Emphasizing "mediumship is not a contagious or mental disease, neither is the spirit a servant," Bandeira pointed out that while mediumship—particularly the remarkable form known as psychic surgery—calls for "nervous characteristics of a special nature", it is not normally associated with mental instability. "Doctors who diagnose 'seeing' or 'speaking' to spirits as mere schizophrenic hallucinations are talking nonsense," he said.

Whilst he agreed that moral factors certainly influenced the quality of mediumship, he could not accept that such factors *governed* the phenomenon.

Commenting on the striking popularity in Brazil of psychic practices grouped under the umbrella of Umbandist centres which today, like Spiritism, claims millions of adherents, Dr Bandeira described Umbanda as a spiritual and psychic amalgam of African "magic", Catholic belief and Kardecism. He said : "It is common practice for a man to belong to Umbanda but to declare himself a Catholic. Here in the state of Guanabara for example, there are now 20,000 Umbanda centres attended by one-fifth of the adult population. Similarly it is estimated that the state of São Paulo contains 18,000 Umbanda centres, and Rio Grande do Sul at least 20,000. Can you wonder that the Catholic Church is sitting up and taking notice? That is why the learned Jesuit researcher Padre Ponciano, has created in Rio an Institute of Psychology where he works with mediums. He is right when he describes mediumship as a divine gift."

Rio de Janeiro, too, has succumbed in a big way to the explosive dynamism of this twentieth-century cult, for the city's remarkable New Year's Eve homage to Yemanja, Brazilian goddess of the sea, annually attracts over half a million people to the city's beaches for midnight ceremonies carried out by over 100,000 white-clad Umbandist midnight celebrants.

No-one, Bandeira assured me, becomes an Umbandist primarily through religious or philosophic convictions. Its attraction lies in the need to seek alleviation of material or spiritual problems. "It has been correctly said," he told me, "that you only enter Umbanda by the door of suffering."

Umbanda's rapid emergence into the sun of widespread acceptance was, in the doctor's view, only one facet of Brazil's astonishing psychic revolution increasingly expressed in an explosion of diverse activities, ranging from Bahia's candomble "priests" in Northern Brazil, whose tribal supremacy required a minimum seven-years' arduous training, to the contrasting types of therapeutic mediumship associated with flourishing Spiritist hospitals which were breaking new ground in mental illness therapy.

Bandeira reminded me that modern medicine could trace back its own forbears to the first witch-doctor who ever brewed a herbal pot-au-feu. Similarly, present-day psychics increasingly demonstrated that "matter is nothing more than condensed energy". He believed the day was near when science itself would attest that what happened in man's material body was reflected in his "peri-spirit", the surviving and semi-material envelope which, Spiritualists affirm, connects man's spirit with the body.

The tumours extracted by psychic surgeons of Brazil and Hawaii, he explained, were not extracted by *physical* cutting but by temporary disintegration of diseased tissue to enable it to be brought to the surface.

In answer to my question : "Why do some patients experience physical pain during psychic surgery?" Bandeira replied that this depended on vibrations, affinity and radiation. There needed to be a harmony of conditions relating to (a) the medium; (b) the patient, and (c) the atmosphere in the room. Psychic surgery, he emphasized, was a delicately balanced psychomental complex. "You may be operating calmly and everything is going well in a wonderful atmosphere, when disharmony erupts, for although we deal and work with unknown forces we cannot yet control them." He instanced a research seance he had attended. During the session a noisy carnival procession had passed by the open-windowed room, completely shattering the psychic harmony of the seance participants. "Everyone began quarrelling and things went haywire until the outside noise and distraction had faded into the distance, after which harmony slowly returned."

He also pointed out that since, as in earthly operations, difficult surgery always requires specialist practitioners the introduction of an unfamiliar "spirit" doctor similarly sometimes causes a degree of disharmony because there had not been opportunity to achieve the same degree of affinity with the medium.

For these and other reasons Dr Bandeira has a high regard for the psychic surgery achievements of his friend Lourival de Freitas. "The way Lourival works is different from the others," he told me. "Lourival has never imposed any limitations upon those who attend his healing sessions, upon where he holds them, or upon how long they last. For these reasons he has frequently come up against very adverse conditions which his guides have got to dominate by gimmicks calculated to build up conviction and confidence in the minds of those present and above all to achieve the delicately balanced complex of psychomental forces necessary to the success of operations in conditions impossible to normal medical techniques."

It was long past midnight when, towards the end of our talk, the doctor predicted: "There are unexplored forces within the human mind so powerful that on the day man discovers them he will be able to achieve an undreamed dominance."

"Do you mean we are on the eve of a Mind revolution?" I asked.

He paused and replied with deliberation: "I would go further and say we are entering a period of cyclic adjustment in humanity's history. We are in a phase of transition and the increasing emergence of supernormal phenomena, spirit healing, psychic surgery and the like, is God's means of reminding man that the world is more than the merely material. I venture to predict that in the age ahead man will eventually make more use of his mind than his body.

"Let us face it, in a very real sense everything is a divine manifestation, otherwise how can you explain Mozart's ability to compose when he was only seven? Why are geniuses the sons of men who are not? And why does a genius in his turn seldom produce children of genius? Such facts contradict the laws of genetics."

Recalling the superb psychic research and experimentation carried out by such nineteenth-century European pioneers as Sir William Crookes, Sir William Barrett, Charles Richet, Baron Schrenk Notzing and Frederic W. H. Myers, Bandeira declared: "Modern spirit healing and countless other spiritual and psychic phenomena contradict all the known canons of official science and nature. They are forcing man to recognize the reality of a supernatural force."

Only the ignorant or the hopelessly prejudiced, he said, could continue to maintain that psychic phenomena were either archaic or to be relegated to the sphere of the primitive and outdated.

Finally, he reminded me that although psychic surgery was still nominally illegal in Brazil, persecution had failed to stem the emergence of a breakthrough in psychic phenomena which was already arousing increasing, albeit controversial, interest among researchers at large and doctors in particular. He revealed that he himself had personal knowledge of nearly a dozen psychic "surgeons" who remained unknown to the public at large. Most of them, he told me, were highly respected citizens. They included a lady in North Brazil, a professor, a magistrate, an army officer and a millionaire.

"Today," said Bandeira, "such gifted psychics have, literally, to operate in secrecy and at considerable personal risk, but I venture to think that a more enlightened science tomorrow will regard it as a privilege to investigate their achievements."

His parting shot was: "Never forget that today's so called 'magic' practices, 'black' or 'white', are primarily based on the power of thought and the repetition of ritual which can canalize and enhance its effects."

9. Lourival: Man and Medium

What manner of man is Lourival de Freitas? Of gypsy lineage he is a man of striking appearance. Tall, pole-slender and aquiline-featured, a crisping mop of grizzled hair, topping a noble forehead of unusual breadth and height, makes him look a decade older than his forty years until he flashes one of his radiant smiles. He has inherited the innate, natural dignity of the pure-blooded gypsy and takes immense pride in the fact that his word is his bond. Shy, sensitive and frequently victim of a precipitate withdrawn moodiness reminiscent of the Highland Celts, he becomes transformed in the company of children and friends he trusts.

He is happiest in his birthplace, the mountain-encircled fishing hamlet of Coroa Grande, nearly two hours' drive south of Rio de Janeiro, where every door is open to him. It is famed for its fine waterfall which has long been a popular centre for weekend "psychic festivals" along its precipitous, wooded course. Lourival was early initiated into occult mysteries. He tells me that as a boy he earned badly needed cruzeiros acting as a water-boy for the weekly invasions of city-dwellers, most of them members of the rapidly-growing Brazilian cult known as Umbandism, which now counts its followers in millions.

Born on October 10, 1929 Lourival was orphaned almost at birth when his parents perished in a fire. He is said to have performed his first "spirit-controlled" operation in trance at the early age of nine, when he cured a stranger of a stomach ulcer. Before this happening he had been found floating unconscious beside the beautiful waterfall near the Porto de Sereia, or Gate of the Siren. When the boy was rescued he told a strange story of a vision which had appeared to him in the form of an impressive figure in shining raiment who had told him clairaudiently (i.e.

a voice had echoed inside his head): "I am Nero." The vision marked the beginning of Lourival's trance mediumship. Lourival also gained a treasury of herbal knowledge from his gypsy grand-mother, said to be of Russian descent, who was locally respected for her own healing powers. I can personally testify that he still frequently supplements his psychic surgery operations with effective herbal remedies.

By the time he was 17 Lourival had already performed many healings in the homes of patients, and even when he served six months' military service in an armoured car unit, he continued to treat soldiers who were ill or who had suffered accidents. Helped by friends, Lourival opened his first healing centre at Rua Antonio Saraiva, Cavalcanti, where he is said to have carried out as many as ten operations daily. Later, at the invitation of a friend he visited Macao, Araparica and Palmeira dos Indios in the state of Alagoas where he continued to treat patients, refusing, as he still does, to accept payment for these services.

A Brazilian journalist, Zora A. O. Seljan, who wrote a profile on Lourival in *Manchete* (October 12, 1968), has told how at this period, in order to earn a living, Lourival began to work in a suburban omnibus company of which he became the manager. Helped by his boss Senhor Abel Fernandes Nunes he opened his second healing centre called the St George Spiritist Centre. Here he worked with teams of mediums.

At this period Lourival's mediumship appeared to have close kinship with Umbandism and it was not until some time later, in a better equipped centre, that Lourival's present form of mediumship evolved. He describes it as the "Roman Cult", because it involves working with a team of spirits headed by Nero. At this third, brick-built centre Lourival held twice-weekly healing sessions in which he carried out upwards of ten operations each session.

At this time Lourival, who had left the bus company, using his indemnity to finance his centre, was earning his living as a salesman of electric irons. Later he became a detective in the police force among whom he still counts many friends.

Lourival's first wife was Zenobia Eustolia Colmo who bore him a son. The marriage ended badly and Zora Seljan has stated that when a sensational court action was brought against Lourival in 1962, charging him with "illegal practice of medicine", the prosecution's two chief witnesses were Lourival's ex-wife and her journalist lover.

Witnesses for the defence included Dr Anselmo de Sa Ribeiro; magistrate Soares Maidonado and Dr Getulio Fonesca Filho. Patients also testified to "cures" they regarded as miraculous and rashly displayed operation scars, thus unwittingly incriminating the man they wished to help. Finally the judge is said to have ordered the accused to demonstrate his powers in a test operation carried out in Caxias, in the house of a man named Valdemar Valduga. The *Manchete* article reported that the patient, formerly a "hopeless case of cancer", was still living. The court, forced to recognize that Lourival was not a charlatan but actually did operate and *did* cure, sentenced him to six months suspended imprisonment which he has never served.

Lourival had to sell his healing centre to pay for the costs in the court case and suffered a breakdown during this unhappy period of his life. Then a friendly invitation from Dr Ademar de Barros, a former governor of São Paulo who was living in exile in Buenos Aires, initiated a far-reaching change in Lourival's life which led to him becoming that rarity among rarities—a peripatetic psychic surgeon who has since become almost as well known outside Brazil as within its borders. During his first visit to a foreign country Lourival is said to have carried out more than fifty operations in Argentina. This in turn led to an invitation from a Brazilian film magnate, which enabled Lourival to visit Los Angeles and California. Here, over a period of $1\frac{1}{2}$ years he carried out another hundred or so operations.

When he returned to Brazil patients and friends in Tijuca raised enough money to buy him a jitney-type taxi (each passenger pays for his seat on shared journeys). Later, another group of grateful patients, headed by General Aristides Leal, arranged for the creation of a trust fund which enables Lourival to maintain a needed car and a pleasantly furnished three-room apartment in a quiet, tree-bowered, residential district in the centre of Rio de Janeiro. When he is in Brazil much of his healing work is carried out at Coroa Grande which he frequently visits. Since 1966, when I met Lourival on his first visit to England, Belgium and France, he has made several return visits to Europe to treat a growing number of patients.

RIDDLING LINKS WITH SHAMANISM

Lourival's complex trance mediumship is of a type unknown in

113

Europe today. When I first saw him operate in a trance in London on June 10, 1966 I wrote that I had met my psychic Eiger; for while I was, and still remain, unshakeably convinced of the validity of what I, and others present, saw that evening, I still cannot begin to explain it.

Yet I was alive to its importance in the field of psychical research, a belief strengthened by subsequent research at the British Museum Reading Room which astonishingly confirmed that this gypsy healer, born in a remote Brazilian coastal hamlet, appears to have mastered in some unknown manner ancient mediumistic rituals involving some of the techniques used by priest-Shamans of Siberian tribes. These rituals are believed by some researchers to be thousands of years old.

I had been guided to this research after reading historical and medical evidence relating to Shamanism published by Dr Andrija Puharich in his copiously documented book *Beyond Telepathy*.

Extraordinary similarities between Shamanistic techniques and some of those used by Lourival de Freitas in the twentieth century emphasize the crucial importance of studying these psychic phenomena with an open mind; for I strongly suspect that such study will possibly yield knowledge which could revolutionize present psychic research vistas and throw fresh light on the psycho-spiritual, folk-medicine traditions and therapy which laid the basis for modern Hippocratic medicine.

Aspects of Lourival's trance mediumship, which aroused controversy in England in 1966 among British Spiritualists, included the healer's use, while in trance, of guitar-accompanied singing and dancing, and drinking undiluted alcoholic beverages such as whisky, and smoking.

To this list of similarities with Asiatic Shamanism can be added Lourival's known preference for holding his healing sessions—sometimes protracted until dawn—in the hours of darkness. He also draws strength and encouragement from the presence of sympathetic spectator-participants, any one of whom may be called upon to assist him during a particular treatment.

All these particular practices appear strange to Europeans, but attested research over decades confirms their sound sense and ancient lineage.

Both Puharich and S. M. Shirokogoroff, a Russian ethnologist who spent years studying paranormal phenomena amongst the Northern Tungus tribes in Siberia, have much to say on the valid reasons for Shamanistic utilization of tobacco and alcohol as aids in tribal trances.

In *Beyond Telepathy*, Puharich tells us:

Shamans use special techniques not only to bring on the state of ecstasy (out-of-body) but to maintain it. Three methods are widely used, namely smoking tobacco, drinking wine or other alcoholic beverages and the use of inebriating mushrooms. However the Shaman usually neither smokes nor drinks before the performance; but it is done when they change spirits and additional excitability is required or when the Shaman is tired.

The smoking may be with an ordinary tobacco pipe, several of which the Shaman may smoke quickly and without interruption. Shirokogoroff has seen five or even six pipes smoked one after the other. The Shaman may also breathe the smoke of resinous conifers, or even incense, the latter being more common among the Tibetan oracles.

The same effect is produced by the taking of alcoholic drinks such as Russian vodka or Chinese wine. A strong person may drink more than a bottle of vodka during his performance.

Puharich also quotes the following passage taken from a sixteenth-century treatise published in Seville relating to the use of tobacco by American Indian priests, to induce trance states:

This plant, which is commonly called tobacco, is a very ancient herb known among the Indians, especially those of New Spain. . . . One of the marvellous things about this plant, which excites the most wonderment, is the manner in which the Indian priests use it. When there is important business among the Indians and the caiques or chiefs of the village think it necessary to consult with the priests, they go to them and state the problem. The priests in their presence take some leaves of the tobacco, throw them on the fire, and receive the smoke of it into their mouths or nostrils, by means of a cane. After taking it they fall down upon the ground as if dead and remain thus, according to the amount of smoke they have taken. When the plant has done its work they recover and give answers, based on the visions and illusions they had while in the trance, and interpret as seems best to them, or as the devil advises them. . . .

Puharich has pointed out that nicotine first excites and then inhibits most of the central nervous system. Similarly, alcohol is a useful aid in enhancing and prolonging trance states since it provides one of the quickest means of energy-absorption.

Shirokogoroff, emphasizing the requirement of great strength to sustain protracted trance activities, tells us that during trance the physical power of a Shaman increases enormously, and his physiological state becomes different from that of normal people. "Ecstasy," he tells us, "requires enormous energy so that all Shamans whom I have observed and who really have been in ecstasy, were unable to move after the performance and were covered with perspiration. The pulse was weak and slow, the breathing was infrequent and shallow."*

Puharich, whose medical knowledge enables him to speak with authority, provides ample pharmacological data relating to the chemical changes in the body which are brought about by smoking and alcohol. He explains how these are aimed at inducing the desired goals of creating the special conditions which liberate the Shaman's "mental self" from the influence of his normal mode of thinking, and which eventually ensure bodily liberation from space and time restrictions.

Puharich confirms that in all Tungus languages Shamanism refers to persons who are said to have "mastered spirits". Shirokogoroff has eloquently described the strict training and nine-day testing of candidate Shamans. The tests include excruciating trial by extremes of heat and cold. Ability to walk on hot coals unharmed, says Shirokogoroff, must be supplemented by a contrasting capacity to general "inner heat". The potential tribal Shaman is required to sit naked in a hole cut in a frozen lake. Water-soaked sheets are thrown around his body and the candidate must then generate enough "Tumo", or body heat, to dry out a succession of frozen sheets. Some, he tells us, have achieved the feat with up to nine and ten successive sheets.

It is a fascinating fact that Lourival has successfully performed fire walking feats, certainly in the early years of his mediumship.

An interesting sidelight on Lourival's strange "stepping-stone"

* S. M. Shirokogoroff, *Psychomental Complex of the Tungus.*

practice, described in detail later, is supplied by Shirokogoroff who asserts that Siberian Shamans frequently experience "an extreme lightness of the body" during deep trance states. He adds, "This feeling is also seemingly communicated to the sick person, for the Manchus assert that when during the performance the Shaman steps on the person lying on the ground, the Shaman is felt to be very light. In fact the feeling of lightness, or in other words, the increase of strength, is a common phenomenon."

He also provides a strange variation of the "sucking" technique effectively resorted to by Lourival in my own case and with other patients. Describing the healing of a sick child by a Tungus Shaman, Shirokogoroff wrote that at one stage "the Shaman sprang upon the child and sucked the body at different parts of the abdomen (especially the navel region, that of the liver, stomach, bladder, appendix and the spleen) so that blood appeared. The Shaman spat out the blood and seemed to be nauseated. After every sucking he cleaned his mouth with wine, but did not vomit."

The Russian researcher also emphasizes the key role of the audience at any Shamanistic seance : "The Shaman with a spirit is no more an ordinary man or relative but is a 'placing' for the spirits : the spirit acts together with the audience (a crowd is desirable) and this is felt by everyone in the audience." Members of the audience, he says, are "both actors and participants".

Emphasizing the importance of a sympathetic attitude on the part of spectators towards the Shaman, Shirokogoroff repeatedly stresses that the influence of negative reactions on a Shamanistic "performance" or seance is great. He warns that in ethnographical records describing such seances, "these demonstrations are often portrayed in a distorted form—as imposture and tricking of the audience." Such an approach, he tells us, "is absolutely erroneous, both from the point of view of the motives of the Shamans and from that of technique", because even the presence of negative or sceptical individuals may "produce confusion in a smooth running performance".

Shirokogoroff also expresses the view that in a Shamanistic session "a permanent current of influences radiated by the Shaman is formed, accepted and intensified by a great number of individuals and sent back to the Shaman for his further excitement. Whether we understand this state of the Shaman—his relations with the audience, mutual hypnosis, suggestion, or even, in a physical form, as peculiar waves—the direct mutual influence of a continuous excitement is such, that the Shaman and the audience become a complex."

For these reasons, he says, the presence of hostility or distrust, is especially dangerous, particularly when foreigners are present who do not understand the process and, fearing to be influenced by it, "assume a hostile attitude of irony or superiority". He remarks that interference by enquirers may "disturb a performance to such a degree that it may turn into a simple ritualistic sequence of acts". Similarly, demonstrative behaviour by the "investigator-observers" may have an equally adverse effect, even though these witnesses might be quite benevolent and well-intentioned.

He points out that if an audience fails to react responsively, the proceedings can degenerate into mere ritualism which will not attain its aim. "Such failures can be actually observed," he says, "and very often public opinion is inclined to see the cause in the Shaman instead of the audience."

While his observations are specifically concerned with Asian Shamanism, they are equally pertinent throughout the whole field of psychic phenomena, especially physical mediumship of the controversial nature demonstrated by Lourival and other Brazilian psychic surgeons, for this obviously presents a *seen* challenge to orthodoxy of any brand—not least those coming within the field of the spiritual and Spiritualist.

Such unfortunately proved to be the case on July 23, 1966 when an invited demonstration of Lourival's mediumship, organized by *Psychic News* and held at the London headquarters of the Spiritualist Association of Great Britain, was unceremoniously brought to an abrupt close. Not surprisingly in the circumstances, the operations carried out were not successful and some critics appeared to suffer a sense of outrage so consuming that wild charges were made with a haste and fervour in inverse proportion to their precariously-based perspicacity.

Veteran Spiritualist, Mrs Ella Sheridan, courageously appealing for "patience and caution in judgement", as opposed to "wholesale condemnation", summed up the sad fiasco and lost opportunity for research in Britain, in an article subsequently printed in *Psychic News* which contained the following pregnant remarks:

The proceedings were so different from anything to which we

are accustomed in this country, or, indeed, in Europe, that many of those present were understandably offended and critical of the methods employed. I must confess that the "set-up" of the theatrical and flamboyant atmosphere did not appeal to me any more than to others. But to condemn anything because it is *different* from what one is used to seems to me to be unscientific and unfair.

She also regretted that a foreigner who had been *invited* to demonstrate, and those who accompanied him, had been discourteously treated in England.

While the evening was a painful experience for all who participated in it, not least the unfortunate guest medium and the patients involved, it served a useful purpose in emphasizing the need at all times for psychic researchers not only to be vigilant, but also *open-minded* in their questing, particularly when viewing techniques alien to their particular culture. Indeed the need for tolerance and humility when approaching psychic mysteries cannot be too strongly stressed if we are to obtain maximum benefit from the seemingly limitless horizons now opening up in the exploding perspectives of psychic and spiritual research.

Certainly the evening had far-reaching and fateful consequences for me, personally, because it led to a welcome invitation to go out to Brazil some months later to study psychic surgery in conditions decidedly more harmonious and less stressful, though equally dramatic and challenging.

10. Human Stepping-Stone and Other Enigmas

Before Joseph Lister, a century ago, ushered in the modern era of "clean surgery", fifty patients out of every 100 subjected to major operations died. Of these, nearly half were victims of gangrene or septicaemia.

Today Western hospitals and operating theatres possess a formidable armoury of defences against post-operative infections. They include such refinements as ultra-sonic washing techniques and sterilization by steam high-vacuum. When necessary, patients can also be temporarily housed in germ-free, totally protective plastic chambers.

A B.B.C. centenary television programme on Lister described him as the man whose revolutionary techniques had "saved more lives than those lost in all the wars of history".

Yet, the toll, though substantially reduced, continues. The same programme surprisingly revealed that "infection after operations" continues to be a menace which probably costs our own Health Service around £6 million yearly.

Viewers were told : "It is reckoned that out of the one-and-a-half million operations carried out in Britain every year, from 2 to 20 per cent result in wound infection."

Additionally the complex hazards associated with the necessary boon of anaesthesia for patients undergoing even comparatively minor operations in modern hospitals have led to recognition of the need for specialized knowledge and training. Today the anaesthetist and his assistants form an indispensable section of all surgical teams, but even in this field of medicine death is no stranger.

Against this background of grim medical facts it is not difficult to picture the horror of the ordinary family doctor or hospital surgeon were he even to find himself witnessing, much less experiencing or participating in any of the run-of-the-mill operations carried out by Lourival and other Brazilian psychic surgeons in medically "impossible" conditions.

Indeed, in any orthodox context the amazing aspect of psychic surgery is not that failures happen, but that *any* successes do. Certainly I can provide no scientific explanation either for the successes *or* the failures. I can only state that apart from the first successful Lourival operation I witnessed in London—and my own —I have witnessed in Brazil more than a score of others just as striking performed by him in the comparatively short periods I have been privileged to watch him at work.

To illustrate the complexity of the problems raised let us take two sample operations, each performed on the same evening in a place, which, for the healer's protection, I shall not identify more closely than to say they took place in the spacious lounge of a home in the tropics. I select them not only because of their intrinsic interest, but also because in both cases I was subseqeuntly able to check that radical improvement had resulted from the treatments I witnessed.

I have additionally chosen them because although they illustrate seemingly contrasted patient reactions *during* treatment, both women later confirmed that no pain had been experienced.

Case one concerned the removal of a large, creamy growth from the eyeball of a seventy-year-old woman, a mulatto. Calling for a standard lamp to be brought nearer to the patient to ensure maximum light for spectators and a photographer present, Lourival plunged a knife up under the woman's eyelid, pressing down upon the eyeball until it almost totally extruded. This brought into view a large growth which almost covered the lower right half of the patient's eye.

Still holding the knife in place the healer then asked a nearby spectator—a retired army general—to wipe off the growth with his finger. The general did so, placing the extracted matter on a cotton-wool swab which was then submerged in a tumbler containing surgical spirit. After swabbing the patient's replaced eye with cotton wool the medium injected a small amount of eye lotion.

The woman remained quite placid throughout the operation and was soon joking and laughing with friends who had accompanied her. When I met her again a month later she reported restored vision in the treated eye.

Case two was even more spectacular, particularly for myself, since I became involuntarily involved. Accompanied by her husband, who held his wife's head and hands steady throughout the ensuing unnerving operation, the patient, an attractive plump brunette in her early thirties, was laid on the floor and surrounded by a large ring of fascinated observers.

Two women helpers unfastened her skirt and bared the stomach area. Understandably nervous and embarrassed, the patient sought to protect her exposed belly by placing her hands upon it. They were repeatedly slapped away by the entranced medium who finally brusquely placed the patient's hands behind her head, indicating that the husband should continue to keep them pinned back.

He then pressed down upon the diseased area and the patient cried out as he plunged scissor points into the flesh at a point he had previously superficially scarred open with a razor blade. The track of the razor was marked by a thin line of oozing blood. Then in a trice the healer had plucked out a large tumour of sickening stench. It was duly photographed.

To my own inwardly panicking dismay I was then ordered by the "surgeon" to cross over to the patient and kneel down by her side. He handed me a knife and instructed me to plunge it into the scarred area. Since I was hesitant to do so, since I was afraid of injuring and causing pain to the unfortunate woman, Lourival then firmly grasped my reluctant hand within his own and forced the knife-blade down and down into what seemed to me an ever yielding chasm of flesh—yet amazingly the flesh wasn't freshly pierced. And much to my surprised relief there was no distressed reaction from the supine patient.

A male helper was then asked to bring over to the medium a bundle of sewing needles, each threaded with ordinary white cotton. I was instructed to hold in my hands each separately threaded "stitch" as de Freitas successively completed his sewing together of the severed flesh out of which the tumour had earlier been extracted.

During the "sewing" one of the needles broke in half. The patient whimpered as each needle plunged through the surface flesh. Finally I held in my nervous hands the threads of nine spaced stitches. To my fresh alarm I was then ordered to pull up the threads tightly until the flesh was visibly raised above normal level. In this position two photographs were taken.

Then came the most astounding interlude of the entire operation. Within a minute or so after the medium had cut away the held threads close to the woman's flesh he demonstrated the complete, inexplicable anaesthesia of the operation area by commanding nearby male spectators—they included the patient's husband and the army general—to step *on* and over her stomach.

Throughout this fantastic and seemingly heartless "game" of human stepping-stones, the patient happily smiled.

When I interviewed her later the same evening, her husband acting as translator, she told me that apart from "discomfort" during the actual stitching, she only remembered a "feeling of pressure" during the stepping-stone incident, but no pain.

I remain utterly baffled as to how this seeming cataleptic anaesthesia was induced. I can only relate that a personal experience of a similar localized "anaesthesia" was vouched for by another man present—a burly bank official. My informant calmly assured me that he, too, had undergone a similar stomach operation performed on him by Lourival a year or two earlier. The man stressed that immediately prior to his operation he had not been able to bear anyone even laying a finger upon his stomach. Yet he too had subsequently undergone the "stepping-stone" experience immediately afterwards. Like the woman I had just interviewed, he too had felt no pain.

Next day the patient's husband telephoned to tell me his wife was feeling well. She was free of pain or post-operative fever. Not surprisingly he added: "I an very happy about the operation." He also told me that he himself had been successfully treated by Lourival for a disease said by his doctors to be inoperable.

I must repeat that during all the "surgery" I saw Lourival perform in varying and extraordinary circumstances, the "operations" were always done in good light and in the presence of witnesses, including close relatives of the patients involved.

On two occasions I actually handled blood-hot tissue immediately after extraction. In each instance I was sickened by its stench. On the first occasion, for hours afterwards, even when I undressed in my bedroom, I seemed to be enveloped by the smell. On the second, although the hostess generously drenched my hands in expensive French perfume, after I had scrubbed them vigorously, the stench similarly lingered for a considerable time.

Perhaps the most dramatic unscheduled operation I saw performed by Lourival in Brazil was the first time I saw him operate on an ear mastoid.

We had motored to Coroa Grande, the fishing hamlet south of Rio de Janeiro, to take midnight photographs of the New Year's Eve Umbandist beach festivals held in honour of Yemanja, Brazilian goddess of the sea.

In the early hours of the morning we adjourned to the still crowded local hotel for refreshments. Word of Lourival's presence had spread throughout the area and about an hour later the patient, a Brazilian sailor, supported by two friends, arrived by car. The man looked ill, staggered and was obviously in pain.

Within minutes he was stretched out on one of the hotel lounge tables which had been hurriedly cleared of glasses and food. A cushion was placed under his head and Lourival, who had gone into trance, commenced treatment by blowing into the affected ear. He then made an incision with scissors in the medically dangerous area immediately below the ear. Bleeding commenced and Lourival quickly extracted convoluted creamy tissue which he placed in my hand. He then stitched the wound, the patient remaining conscious throughout. Within half an hour the formerly suffering patient, now free of pain and smiling happily, joined others dancing to a jazz melody played on a gramophone. Only one ban was imposed by Lourival. He told the patient he must not drink any alcohol for the next twenty-four hours.

The scope and skill of Lourival's psychic surgery is also attested in the following striking personal testimony written by Cleusa de Penaforte, a well-known Brazilian opera singer. The singer swore to the truth of her signed testimony in the presence of a Rio de Janeiro public notary. Here is a translation of her statement, dated October 10, 1964.

At 00.30 in the morning of August 13, 1963, I received a telephoned invitation from Senhora Adelita M. Ferreira to meet Sr Lourival de Freitas about whom I had heard the most remarkable things. I went to the home of Mrs Cloris Smith, where I had witnessed events which greatly impressed me since they seemed to defy known physical laws as well as the laws of medicine.

I saw Sr Lourival de Freitas, the remarkable medium, under

control of his Spirit Guide, who alleges to be the great Nero, the powerful Roman Emperor, perform an operation on the body of my hostess for the removal of two so-called "bicos de papagaio" (spinal calcifications popularly termed parrot's beaks).

This operation was performed in the most extraordinary manner. The patient lay down calmly. A few centimetres of blood, taken from one of the spectators present, without regard to blood type, were injected into her. The needle and syringe had not been previously boiled, neither had any of the instruments or materials used in the operation, such as scissors, penknife, kitchen knife, tweezers, etc. Nothing was sterilized in any way, indeed on a subsequent occasion I watched this same marvellous medium clean the penknife on the sole of his shoe, saying that he was sterilizing it. He then used it for another operation I witnessed.

I noticed with astonishment that the patient kept up a conversation during the operation, while the "parrot's beaks" were being extracted. The operation was rapidly and brilliantly performed, as were so many others that I have since been able to witness, performed on well known people in political and social circles.

Mrs C. S., who had previously suffered dreadful pain, got up after the two incisions had been stitched and at the command of the extraordinary spirit guide, Nero, proceeded to do some violent gymnastics—which, after any ordinary operation, would have been quite impossible. I observed, as did her family, that these caused her no pain.

Finally, I declare that after this I saw other marvellous operations carried out by the genius of charity and love. His greatest originality is his ability to do all these things in a highly artistic manner. *I myself had the pleasure of being operated on by him a week before my concert at the International Festival of Music*, where I was to sing with the Symphonic Orchestra and a chorus of 80 voices, the famous Cantata of Brahms for contralto and male choir.

Immediately after operating on my throat, when he removed my spongy tonsils, during which I felt absolutely no pain whatsoever, he commanded me to sing. I found that I was able to sing with the greatest ease the fourth act from "Aida" by Verdi. As I am an opera singer at Rio de Janeiro, São Paulo, Rio

Grande do Sul, Belo Horizonte, having also sung with the Paris opera company and others, I have been able to help Nero through my singing in his wonderful work.

I have seen him perform operations for cancer, cataract, throat, slipped disc, ulcer and other marvels, all carried out within minutes.*

The work of this fine medium is extraordinary. He is truly a strange mystic. Nero, through Lourival de Freitas, is and will remain an enigma to mankind. Researchers, philosophers and occult mystics will not easily analyse him. He is the unexpected who defies the laws of science with the material proofs of his achievements. We must render our thanks to the powers of this singular man who has saved so many lives and brings happiness to so many.

DEATH OF A COW

During my stay in Brazil I also had the good fortune to witness another riddling aspect of Lourival's many-faceted psychic powers used on this occasion, not to prolong life, but to bring to a speedy, merciful end an animal's unendurable suffering. It was for me a most moving example of unorthodox euthanasia without the aid of drugs or the customary bullet.

I witnessed this fantastic little Bethlehem "in reverse" when Lourival was asked to give aid to an eight-year-old pedigree Guernsey cow suffering over a strangulated birth. It was her fifth calf.

It happened on the evening of December 13 in a mountain valley smallholding, some eighty miles distant from Rio. During dinner in Rio he had received an emergency call from Francisco, the hardworking young farmer of German descent who looked after the rural property. He had telephoned in some distress to report that the calf had come feet first and the head was too large to allow passage. Francis had been a helpless witness to the

* She gives details of where her throat operation was performed, and names of other successfully treated patients for tumour of the prostate (his own doctor assisted the medium); tracoma (specialists seen in Brazil, London and Madrid had been unable to do anything); cancer in the genital organs to a named woman.

cow's 15-hour ordeal, which had included unsuccessful "bleeding" by two veterinary surgeons called in. They had recommended that the animal should be destroyed.

By good fortune Lourival was present as a guest at dinner. Within minutes of the telephone call we were all on our way by car to the farm. When we arrived around 10 p.m. we found the cow—a beautiful animal with heartrending lustrous brown eyes— lying on her side in a semi-open thatched byre, her head resting on straw. She uttered continuous pitiful moans. From her uterus two of the calf's legs extended grotesquely, one of them broken at the knee joint as a result of earlier manhandling. When he set eyes on her Lourival had shaken his head over her plight. After ordering that the farmhands be sent out of the byre he became entranced. Calling for a pad and pen he began to draw a diagram of the cow's womb, muttering to himself as he marked different sections. A pail of water was brought into the byre and after plunging his hand and arm into the cow's uterus he told us the calf had died in the imprisoning womb. Tetanus, he said, had already set in. But I noticed with relief that although at one point he had pulled the cow right around, using the calf's dangling legs as a lever, the animal had ceased to groan. At intervals he washed his hands, sipped whisky and smoked a cigarette.

Appearing to abandon the idea of trying to save the cow by removing the calf, he then began timing some unseen process, partly by checking with his wristwatch, which he had not removed during his earlier examination, and partly by checking off with his fingers. He seemed to be in touch with unseen forces and awaiting a certain signal. At all times, intensely, compassionately intent upon the quietly prone animal, he appeared to be able, by merely raising his hand, to control her slightest movement, for suddenly, as if in obedience to his will, she raised her head and silently began —mouth open and tongue slightly extended as if to suck in maximum air—to make weaving, snake-like movements in ever widening arcs. At maximum stretch her jaw hit a post near me with some force, but no sound came from her; the eyes were fixed and already slightly receding into her head. Then movement ceased as her head came to rest against a light fencing which separated the byre from a small pen containing two piglets. One of them repeatedly tried to reach over the barrier, then poig- nantly tried to muzzle the dying animal with its own little snout pushed under the base of the barrier. It was so damned human you could swear the cow understood its neighbourly attempt to comfort. For myself, I don't mind confessing that as I watched the slender figure of the man, seated on an upturned box, I prayed hard for a speedy end to the suffering we were helplessly watching. Then Lourival, as if he had received an awaited signal, stood up. After a final glance at his watch he gave the exhausted animal its last human salutation in the form of encouraging claps and strokes along her back, neck, horns and brow. With his knuckle, he then appeared to make the sign of a cross at a point just behind the horns. There was the briefest responding fall back of the cow's head. Her tongue extruded, discoloured and limp. It was all over.

A minute or two later, holding a lighted candle for which he had asked, he voiced a brief noble invocation. It asked God's pardon for the mercy killing granted in the name of love, paid homage to death's liberation and expressed a plea for redemptive aid upon all suffering life.

11. Psychic Surgery in N.W. London

When Lourival de Freitas arrived in London in August, 1969, stopping off on his way to Belgium to see patients, an English friend organized a "welcome back" party in his honour. As always, at any gathering which centres on this astonishing man, guests included former patients who, like myself, had benefited from his healing ministrations, and others, brought by friends, who hoped they, too, might receive similar spirit-inspired aid. In the earlier hours of the evening the gay gathering, entertained with Brazilian music and light refreshments, was indistinguishable from any conventional party of friends, old and new.

When Lourival and his party, which included his young Brazilian wife Aparecida and his baby daughter Dulandula, arrived around 9.30 they mingled with the guests who included devoted Brazilian friends, students, young artists and a tidy sprinkling of professional people who numbered in their ranks psychiatrists, two professors and a learned linguist. Although the majority of guests present could be termed newcomers to the field of paranormal phenomena, goodwill and open-minded interest prevailed throughout the evening. This was particularly noticeable during the memorable events which followed when Lourival eventually became entranced by his control, Nero.

Of the four treatments I was privileged to witness at close quarters, only two of them came within the specific category of psychic surgery. The instruments used by the entranced medium comprised a steel-handled knife, a razor-blade and scissors. Both patients expressed their gratitude for beneficial results.

The first poignant, non-surgical treatment which undoubtedly intensified the already existing feeling of goodwill towards the medium, was given to a pretty, five-year-old girl who was deaf and dumb. She had been brought by her adoptive parents who told Lourival that medical specialists had been unable so far to alleviate her tragic plight, since no physical defect had been found to account for her total deafness which had not been discovered until the child was turned two years old. Doctors were of the opinion that it was a nerve deafness, probably inherited, but no confirmatory information could be given to the Brazilian healer about the medical history of the child's parents whose whereabouts were not known.

Lourival, after praising the devotion shown to the child by her adoptive parents, commented on the difficulties presented by the absence of information linking with the child's natural parents, but said he would attempt to influence the child's "peri-spirit" by means of musical sound and rhythm. He quickly won the playful child's confidence and she was lifted up on to a bed where he and a Brazilian friend held her protectively. Lourival then asked a young Belgian singer present to "sing with all his might" an unaccompanied operatic aria. The assembled company were also asked to concentrate on helping both child and singer, and silence fell upon the room as the fine tenor voice soared and sank in the golden notes of a famous Wagner aria.

The effect upon the child was astonishing. Immediately she lost her restless vivacity and very quickly sank into a serene slumber, oblivious of scores of watching eyes. As the song progressed she gradually slid down from the bed, away from the protective arms which held her, to the floor where she continued to sleep soundly, stretched out between our crowding feet.

The aria was followed by a lively song played on the guitar by Lourival who was still in trance. It was noticed that the music increasingly seemed to penetrate the sleeping child's subconscious mind. Still asleep, she began to move her arms and legs vigorously in rhythmic harmony with the beat of the music. When she awoke she was greeted by her delighted parents and soon flung herself happily into the arms of the healer.

No immediate or decisive results had been promised as a result of the treatment but the child's "father" in subsequent reports given to the healer said that from the day after her treatment there was a marked beneficial psychological improvement in the child's attitude and behaviour. Formerly she had always been a highly-strung, nervy child; now she had become unusually happy and calm. The improvement had also been commented upon by teachers at her school.

The adoptive father, a victim of duodenal ulcers, who later that evening underwent a "spirit" operation which had involved threaded needles being passed through his flesh in the stomach area, had also happily reported during the week following that he had become free of pain, was able to eat foods formerly forbidden to him and "felt very well".

The first traditional-type "psychic surgery" operation turned out to be a visually unnerving eye operation carried out on one of my friends, Mr Gordon Creighton, a middle-aged linguist and scholar. He had earlier asked Lourival whether he could alleviate a long-standing sinus affliction. The patient had not mentioned that he was also troubled by a deterioration in his eyesight, but the healer's preliminary examination had established what he described as a developing condition of glaucoma in the left eye. The examination was carried out in an adjoining bedroom but the patient was brought back into the centre of the crowded sitting-room for the subsequent "psychic surgery".

Many present gasped with dismay when they saw Lourival take up a sharp steel knife, thrust the patient's head backwards and insert the knife blade forcefully under the patient's eyelid and apparently into the tissue above the eye. Within seconds the healer had withdrawn the knife and placed into the nerveless hand of the patient's nearby watching wife a substance extracted from the eye.

The patient, who merely described his seemingly harrowing experience as "uncomfortable", was placed in a fireside armchair where he remained with eyes closed for a time. There was no bleeding and when I telephoned my friend next day he cheerfully told me his sight in both eyes had improved. Nine months later he confirmed that no deterioration in the left eye had subsequently taken place.

The next operation was equally dramatic, and successful. The patient on this occasion was a charming young Norwegian ballet dancer who had been unable to follow her career for two years, following a spinal disc injury sustained in over-zealous, back-straightening dance exercises.

Both the young patient and her mother told me that while doctors had been able to treat the disc displacement, they had been baffled by the patient's recurring bouts of excruciating spinal pain which they attributed to some form of pressure for which they were unable to diagnose the cause. For two years she had received treatments in Norwegian, Danish and English hospitals, but the pain continued. The girl told me : "I used to scream during the attacks."

I was particularly interested in the psychic surgery techniques used in this back operation which reminded me in some respects of my own earlier operation, carried out by Lourival in December 1966 to alleviate a very different medical condition—bronchiectasis.

The medium first asked for a razor blade with which he deeply scarred open an arc of flesh about five to six inches long on the girl's back. Then he asked for a pair of scissors which he dug into the wound in order to cut more deeply into the flesh.

The young dancer was then placed in a reclining position, face downwards on a settee, with the lower half of her body and legs on the floor. In this position a glass was placed on top of the bloodied wound. The patient appeared to have fallen into a deep sleep which lasted for the duration of the operation. Lourival left her unattended for a short while to attend to earlier patients in an adjoining room, after ordering that no-one should go near her and so disturb what was described as an "ectoplasmic current" which apparently flowed from two spectators, a man and a woman, who had suddenly become entranced. When Lourival returned he removed the glass and manipulated the bloodied scar with his hands. Then he placed his mouth over the wound and began to suck with considerable force. Within seconds he had sucked out a small piece of whitish tissue. As the spectators crowded round to examine it the girl rose to her feet, none the worse for her experience.

Then Lourival asked for a cotton-threaded needle which he drew through the two lips of the cut flesh in the centre of the operation scar until they met. Afterwards he pulled out the thread. Then after he had lightly wiped away bloodstains from the wound, using a small ball of medicated cotton wool I had myself purchased earlier that day, astonished spectators perceived that the formerly blood-spouting wound had mysteriously closed to a pencil-thin red scar.

The laughing happy young patient was then instructed to "perform the most difficult arm exercises you know". She did so with graceful ease and soon afterwards joined Lourival in a happy victory dance. When I congratulated her later she told me she was quite pain free. She said she had felt nothing during the "operation" apart from a slight "nip", possibly when the open stitch was made with the needle.

There were two "thank you" postscripts to her "spirit" operation. The first took the form of a celebration party given by the patient's grateful parents in their home in Lourival's honour. The second was a profoundly moving letter sent by the patient to Lourival, which I was privileged to read. Written in English, with quaint turns of phrase, the girl thanked Nero for having "released me from suffering" and brought back renewed life which "for a long time has been paralysed by pain". She wrote: "I have been in a storm. And suddenly all is quiet. I have been in a hell. And finally someone has lifted me up, and brought me to a place of security and warmth. . . . When you were singing, it doesn't matter who believes it or not, I remember looking into your eyes and we were both laughing. In that moment I really realized I was cured, and that you knew what had happened was too great to be vocally explained and that just those who are open and aware of miracle will believe it by my few words 'something was in me and now it is gone!' "

12. Arigó

Up to the time of his death in a car crash on January 11, 1971, José Pedro de Freitas,* affectionately known to millions by his nickname "Arigó", which can be roughly translated as meaning a good guy, enjoyed a popularity said to have rivalled that of another fellow Brazilian, the famous footballer Pelé.

Twice-jailed psychic surgeon and spirit leader, Arigó was a native of the picturesque hill town of Congonhas do Campo in the mountainous iron ore mining region of the state of Minas Gerais.

His first imprisonment took place in 1958 for the "crime" of illegal practice of medicine. Although a Brazilian doctor had eloquently testified in court that his own life had been saved by Arigó's timely, unpaid ministrations, the healer was sentenced to a two and a half years' prison term. He did not complete it, thanks to a surprise pardon later granted by Kubitschek, a former President of Brazil. Rumour has it that Arigó had earlier successfully treated a member of Kubitschek's own family.

The healer's second collision with the law occurred in 1961. Investigations had laggardly dragged on for some three years until, on November 20, 1964, Marcio Aristeu Monteiro de Barros, a county judge, passed sentence of sixteen months' imprisonment. Pedro McGregor, in his biographical chapter "Surgeon of the Rusty Knife",† quotes the following extract from the sententious antediluvian judgement:

Witchcraft is punished to safeguard the individual and the public well-being. The man who, without being a doctor,

* No relation to Lourival.
† *The Moon and Two Mountains* by Pedro McGregor.

determines the nature of a sickness or illness by their symptoms: who, without being a doctor, makes operations: who, claiming to be in the "control" of a "spirit", in trance, prescribes or operates, or supplies herbs: who uses "passes", attitudes, postures, words, prayers, exorcisms or any other means to facilitate childbirths, cure a rebellious cough, snake bites, cancer, lower fever, tuberculosis, haemorrhage, cataracts, deafness, etcetera—this citizen represents a tremendous danger to the health of an undetermined number of people whose custody unquestionably is entrusted upon the state.

Once again Arigó found himself behind bars. Once again, following mass protests, demonstrations in Brazil and international petitions organized in many countries inside and outside Latin America, Arigó was released on parole months before his time was up. Even during his imprisonment, I was told, his cell had become a Mecca for sick suppliants.

It was on an improvised "screen"—the white-painted wall of a thirteenth-floor room in a São Paulo skyscraper hotel—that I first saw a colour film of Arigó's amazing "psychic surgery". It was shown to me by Jorge Rizzini, a courageous writer who is himself a convinced Spiritist.

The film I saw on that January evening in 1967 had already made history in the stormy annals of Brazil's century of psychic progress, for Rizzini's tireless campaigning throughout the subcontinent and in neighbouring countries had undoubtedly played a significant role in helping to secure Arigó's early release "on parole" before the completion of his second prison sentence.

His film certainly made a lasting impression on me and an even sharper impact on my student translator. Opening shots of this colour film show the entranced medium puncturing and draining the swollen testicles of a Brazilian peasant. Although the patient appeared placid the gory shots markedly affected my young friend. After rushing across to an open window "for air", he explained, he fled out of the room, excusing his precipitate exit on the grounds of "the undue heat of the room". I sympathized, for had I myself not been forearmed and fortified by having earlier witnessed similarly sensational trance feats during my study of the mediumship of Lourival de Freitas, I doubt whether I could have watched the film through to its conclusion.

I had the good fortune to meet Rizzini again a week later in Belo Horizonte, capital of the state of Minas Gerais. He was planning to make a second documentary film of José Arigó at work, for showing on his São Paulo television programme, and we motored to Congonhas accompanied by mutual friends, Professor Roberto Carneiro and his delightful wife Jilda.

Leaving Belo Horizonte around daybreak we drove across the mountains at sunrise, arriving at Arigó's "Spiritual Centre of Jesus Nazarene" shortly before 8 a.m. Sited in a narrow cobbled street in the heart of the picturesque colonial town we found it already crowded with its first daily influx of patients.

From 6 a.m. onwards on weekdays, interrupted only in the afternoons when Arigó went off to attend to his own affairs, returning in the late afternoon to attend to another tidal wave of patients, they filled the ranged wooden benches in the main hall of the decrepit, paint-peeling building. Young and old, of every nationality and shade of human pigment, the medical discards and the disconsolate, many silent in their personal despairs, others made vociferous in a shared last hope, the well-dressed and the elegant sat shoulder to shoulder with cripples, beggars, distracted ancients and young children. In the background, whenever a helper remembered to put on a record, a cracked gramophone of ancient vintage provided music.

Handwritten slogans and admonitions, interspersed by portraits of Jesus and a wall crucifix, decorated the time-grimed, lime-washed walls at the time of my visit. Part of the ceiling had broken away and its gaping hole reaching to the rafters had been roughly patched with green-painted wood trellising, festooned with cobwebs and dust. Wall inscriptions—some of them signed "Arigó", others bearing the name of his famous spirit "control", Dr Fritz—were blunt: AVOID ALCOHOL, TINNED FOODS, PORK, ONIONS AND SMOKING. Dr Fritz. HEALING SESSIONS AND SPIRITUAL ADVICE AT THIS CENTRE FROM 8 MONDAYS TO FRIDAYS ANYONE WHO WISHES. IT IS FORBIDDEN TO ASK FOR DONATIONS IN THIS HOUSE. THE SPIRITISM OF KARDEC WITHOUT UMBANDA OR MACUMBAS. HAVE FAITH, JESUS WILL CURE.

In the winter of 1967, Arigó, still under the duress of parole, was unable to carry out any of the more sensational psychic surgery operations which had won him fame, but during the two days we spent at Congonhas we were privileged not only to witness and photograph startling eye treatments which he humorously described as "examinations", but also to "feel for ourselves" the depth of the knife's penetration into the bony area of eyebrow tissue. In no single case did any of us either observe, or afterwards receive from the patients concerned, any complaints of pain or infection.

Furthermore, although it was stressed that we had only witnessed eye *examinations,* three patients I interviewed through my translator told me their sight had radically improved.

The first, a Rio gem merchant in his sixties, was a victim of glaucoma, a condition which had been confirmed by doctors he had seen both in London and Barcelona. "I got very ill," he told me. "Every effort I made to have an operation in London failed. Every doctor I visited said they could do nothing for me. When I arrived in Congonhas from Europe ten days ago, Dr Fritz told me I had just come in time. It was almost too late." Looking a very happy man indeed he confirmed that after the second "examination" sight had been restored in both eyes.

The second patient, Senhora Elvira Floriano Coasta Silva, lived in Santo Andres, near the city of São Paulo. She told me she had made the long overnight journey to Congonhas by bus. "Sixteen years ago", she said, "the sight in my left eye started to become weak and increasingly painful. My doctor could only prescribe glasses and eventually I lost my sight in that eye. When I arrived here this morning, before Dr Fritz treated me, I could not read any of these wall notices. Now I can." When I asked her if she had felt any pain when the sharp-pointed knife had been jabbed so deeply into the eye socket, she replied : "Not pain. I'm very glad I came. You can see for yourself there is no bruise."

The third patient, a retired chemist, told me he was a Spiritist. His oculist had diagnosed a retina thrombosis in the left eye and had advised against an operation. He, too, confirmed that sight in this affected eye had improved after the "demonstration" I had witnessed. He said he had only felt "a moment's prick" when the knife was initially inserted.

Jorge Rizzini, Pedro McGregor, Joao Martins and Moacyr Jorge are only a handful among many journalists who have all testified to striking evidence given by medical witnesses privileged to watch the Arigó-Dr Fritz partnership at work. Dr Ary Lex, a São Paulo University lecturer on surgery, is one of many medical witnesses who have praised Arigó's fantastic "surgery" on Brazilian television programmes. Lex, like others, said that although he had been initially sceptical, the surgery he had witnessed had been undeniably genuine. Operations he described included cyst drainage without normal surgical preparations, and the removal of a non-malignant tumour from a woman's arm without cutting open the flesh. "He sort of rubbed the skin with the back of his scalpel until it opened up," Lex reported. "He then squeezed the lipoma with his fingers and it came out whole."

In another operation described by Lex as spectacular and astounding, he told how Arigó, during an eye operation, had inserted scissors, cut the tissue and when it bled "he just passed a piece of ordinary cotton wool over it and produced immediate haemostasis" (cessation of bleeding). He added that Arigó had "cleaned" his scalpel by violently rubbing it on the head of another distinguished medical witness present, Professor Accorsi. The professor, he said, had felt no discomfort and no infection had resulted. Lex urged scientific study of the medium.

Another São Paulo medical specialist, Dr José Hortencia de Medeiros Sobrinho, had accompanied a friend when the latter in despair had taken his 28-year-old Polish wife, a hopeless cancer case, to see Arigó. Before treatment the woman's condition had been "desperate". The first treatment had consisted in "Dr Fritz" prescribing several medicines in unusually high dosages. Dr Sobrinho said: "To our great surprise, after the first week, her improvement was so marked that she was able to get up and walk around." After a third visit she had been pronounced "cured". Dr Sobrinho testified that this was later confirmed when a hospital doctor had "found only a few fibroids in the woman's abdomen, but no tumour".

More and more in recent years, however, owing not only to the unending flood of patients but also legal harrying, healing-by-prescription necessarily increasingly dominated at Arigó's healing centre, where hundreds of sick suppliants were seen daily.

After a short introductory homily from Arigó, pungent and shot with humour about human failings, the endless snaking line of patients began to file, shoulder to shoulder, through an anteroom into his tiny consulting room where he sat at an ink-stained desk ludicrously dwarfed by his bulk. Diagnosis and prescriptions—the latter frequently long and complicated—were completed at a supernormal speed, averaging nearly one a minute. During the period I was privileged to sit by his side as patient after patient was dealt with, I was astonished to note that even as each stranger reached his desk, and before the medium had barely glanced up, he had begun to write out the prescription, in a kind of medical shorthand, later transcribed and typed for the patient by Arigó's assistant in a neighbouring room.

Faced with the self-pitying or self-indulgent, Arigó could be bluntly brusque, telling them "Go home" or "You eat and sleep too much". On one occasion when a Brazilian authoress, as a trick test, had sent her chauffeur to stand in line, he was cursorily dismissed: "What did you come here for? Go away! Give your place to those who need it." But to those really ill compassion was unfailing. When he was faced with a hopeless case Arigó would quietly write out a prescription, but would frequently take accompanying relatives aside and explain to them that death would be inevitable.

The memory I can never forget from my own eyewitness experience was that of a tall, elderly Brazilian in that unending queue. Learning that I was a foreign journalist who had come to study Arigó, he broke file to tell me—tears streaming down his face—of the debt of gratitude he owed to "Dr Fritz" whose prescription had cured his mother of cancer some years earlier. He told me: "Yet she had been given up by her doctor as a hopeless case with only a short time left to her."

Congonhas do Campo has long been famous not only for the beauty of its baroque churches but above all for the works of a sculptor, Antonio Francisco Lisboa, who lived there in the early part of the nineteenth century. An epileptic crippled in both hands and feet, Lisboa, like Arigó, is better known by his nickname "Aleijadinho", which means the "little cripple". Incredibly, the artist, who devised primitive instruments tied to his arms after he had been carried to the site of his work, created sculptures of genius. His finest series of soapstone statues of the Twelve Apostles are the glory of the beautiful church which crowns the mountain at the foot of which the little town nestles.

Pedro McGregor tells us: "Today, Congonhas do Campo has two stars: Aleijadinho and Arigó. Some come to see one; some the other. The smart ones go to see both. But those who go to see Arigó cannot fail also to experience Aleijadinho—not his work, not the Twelve Apostles created here on earth, but what he does on the spiritual plane. For the spirit of the sculptor is in fact 'in charge' of all the work done through Arigó by 'Dr Fritz' and his astral colleagues : all the cures, all the operations are carried out under his spiritual 'direction'."

It is a beautiful story which deserves to be true. I only know that the work of healing which went on daily in the modest building at the foot of the hill dwarfed in majesty all the costly treasures which crowded the gilded interiors of the baroque churches above it. Truly, the healing centre of "Jesus Nazareno" was well-named.

What manner of man *was* José Arigó? It is a question which can hardly be answered adequately in the singular, for the genius of Arigó—as with other psychic surgeons and many spiritual healers—rested in the fact that whatever alternative explanations might be proffered or preferred by the orthodox and the sceptic, remarkable personality changes manifested whenever they were overshadowed by "spirit" controls.

Arigó, the man, was built like a boxer, rustic in speech, placid, genial, good-natured and generous; a family man who long fought fearlessly for the underdog. Born into a conventional, comfortably-off farming family of staunch Catholics, Arigó, easy-going and unambitious, preferred farm life in his early youth. A month before his twenty-sixth birthday in 1944 he married a local girl, and six sons resulted.

To maintain his growing family he went to work in one of the iron-ore mines in which this mountainous district abounds. Rising at 3 a.m. he had to walk eight miles to his work. Pay was so poor that in the early years of the marriage his wife became a seamstress to help make ends meet. Arigó began to speak out against the insufferable conditions and formed a local union branch of which he was elected president. After leading them in a strike he was sacked and blacklisted for militancy. Jobless and a family out-cast he was eventually financed by a family loan and opened a bar and restaurant. It became very popular and he was finally able to buy land and live in what Pedro McGregor and others have described as a fine home. But McGregor has described Arigó as a man unable to say "No" to requests for help. After being badly let down by a fly-by-night politician the café was closed.

Meanwhile, his practical problems had been enhanced by a recurrence of strange happenings in his personal life which disturbed him greatly. They concerned supernormal events. Arigó also became increasingly troubled by fainting fits for which doctors could find no physical cause. It was the commencement of his mediumship. McGregor's account of this period states that night after night Arigó became troubled by the appearance in his bedroom of a bald, fat-bellied man who told him in German-accented Portuguese: "You will cure many." Arigó's alarmed wife begged him to see a doctor. A priest was also called in to exorcize "the devil". The visitations continued and Arigó's "faints" increased.

Then came the event which radically changed the whole course of Arigó's life, bringing him an unsought fame. It concerned an unscheduled operation upon a well-known Brazilian Senator, Lucio Bittencourt, victim of carcinoma of the colon. Many differing versions of this event have been published but the following researched account is based on a transcript taken from my shorthand notes when I attended a remarkable lecture given at Centre House Community, London on July 11, 1968. It was vouched for by Dr Andrija Puharich, the well-known New York neurologist whose medical and psychic researches in the post-war decades have culminated in a still continuing intensive depth study into Arigó's astonishing psychic gifts, expressed in his uncannily accurate diagnostic abilities and psychic surgery operations.

Arigó's unsought leap into the headlines had been prefaced by a journey to Belo Horizonte to pay family taxes. He had stayed in a small pension in the county capital where one of the guests was Lucio Bittencourt. Bittencourt, with whom Puharich later checked the following facts when he first met him in 1963, said he had been wakened between 3 and 4 a.m. by a knock on his bedroom door.

When he opened the door he had found a stranger, standing with a razor in his hand. He appeared to be in a sleep-walking state. The man had entered the room and told the dumbfounded Bittencourt to lie down on the bed. He had then pulled up the Senator's pyjama jacket and carved him open. Bittencourt had told Puharich he felt no pain and the whole thing had seemed to take only a matter of minutes. The stranger had opened up the abdominal wall, went in with the razor and produced a section of the victim's colon—a tumour which he dropped on the bed. Bittencourt had then fallen asleep and woken at 8.30 a.m. It was only when he saw blood spattered over the bed, surveyed his torn, blood-stained pyjamas and found the tumour that, in the words of Puharich, "he remembered what had happened and got panicky".

The Senator had had a medical check up only a few weeks

earlier. Cancer of the larger intestine had been diagnosed and he was scheduled for surgery. Bittencourt quickly recovered from his nocturnal operation and puzzled doctors later confirmed that a tumour had indeed been removed. He told everyone "this crazy story" of the man who had slit him open. Inquiries were made as to who had done it and when Arigó was brought before Bittencourt the Senator identified him as the man who had operated. Arigó angrily denied it, but since Bittencourt got well no charges were ever brought. Puharich said the Senator had remained a loyal friend of Arigó, up to the time of his death in 1967 when he died in an aeroplane accident.

Another sensational "operation" happened two months later in Arigó's home town when he had visited a woman dying of an abdominal tumour. Arigó had been sitting at the woman's bedside, together with other relatives and neighbours, when he suddenly jumped up and brought a butcher's knife from the kitchen. Cutting the dying woman open in front of the horrified witnesses he had brought out a uterine tumour weighing 14 lbs. He then ran out of the house. Puharich told us: "I personally talked to the woman years later. She is still alive."

He also told of the subsequent interest taken in Arigó in those early years of his psychic healing by priests in the local Basilica monastery. Arigó himself was a devout Roman Catholic. For five years he was only allowed to heal under the supervision of the monks who had sought to curb Spiritist heresies. The growing conflict between the realities of his mediumistic activities and the monks' strictures regarding "evil spirits" had finally become insupportable and Arigó took a major decision.

Puharich said: "He gave up the monks. Now he has nothing to do with Roman Catholicism except that he keeps up a lovely dialogue with the local priest. It is quite an amusing 'Don Camillo' situation."

Puharich revealed that he himself had first become aware of Arigó's existence "quite by accident" in 1963 when he had visited Brazil on a very contrasting mission connected with the U.S. National Aeronautics and Space Agency. Scientists, he said, were becoming increasingly interested in the mysterious nature of the force of gravity. Could there be such a thing as anti-gravity? He had been sent to Brazil to investigate reports of a psychical medium who lived near the international airport of São Paulo and who was said to be capable of levitating heavy objects by merely staring at them. He had hoped to be given permission to study this man's mediumship but had failed to win the confidence of the well-meaning Spiritists who surrounded him and who were suspicious of American scientists. Then a Professor of Medicine in Rio de Janeiro had told him about Arigó's psychic surgery operations and his own first-hand experiences. At the time Puharich confessed he had doubted his friend's sanity, but thought that since he had come so far he might as well investigate. He journeyed to Congonhas do Campo and spent ten days observing Arigó at work. "What I saw during that time," he said, "fully corroborated what my friend had told me. Eventually I reached a point of true incredulity. I could not believe what I was seeing, so I asked Arigó to operate on me, to remove a fatty tumour on my right arm."

Puharich said that if this comparatively minor operation had been carried out in a hospital, it would have taken between 15 and 20 minutes to perform. Arigó, however, without even sterilizing his knife, or worrying about anaesthetizing his patient, had deftly removed the tumour in around five seconds. "I felt something wet in my hand," said the doctor, "and there was the tumour. I figured I had been defrauded. It happened so fast and I had not even felt anything. All had gone past me like something at high velocity. And remember he was using a dirty knife on my unwashed arm. How, then, could he control bacterial infection? He didn't use any antibiotics, yet my arm healed with no complications. And a film taken at the time bore witness to what had happened."

Puharich had become hooked. Here was an untrained, medically ignorant, ex-tin miner breaking all the rules of orthodox surgery in a fantastic manner and—what was even more unbelievable—getting away with it. For although, like the medical fraternity at large, Arigó was no stranger to failure, no-one had ever successfully brought any charge that the Congonhas healer's ministrations had proved lethal to a patient, or even demonstrably harmful. Puharich knew that if Arigó, as he had now successively witnessed, could seemingly set aside the normal hazards of surgery even when carried out in near-ideal operative conditions, then he must be obeying other laws of nature equally, or perhaps more, cogent than those already known to science. Here indeed was an outsize medical riddle, an enigma which cried out to be scientifically investigated. Was this perhaps the intended purpose of so-called "psychic surgery"? If so Puharich was the right researcher at the right spot, for his several published medical research contributions, widely esteemed by doctor colleagues, eloquently testify that he is not a man to flinch from any challenge presented to his professional attention. At New York University he became a member of a team of specialists who are working on producing a mechanical heart for transplants. He is also associated with a remarkable breakthrough in research connected with deafness.

Since that first visit he returned to Congonhas many times. In May, 1968, accompanied by a team of six doctors and eight other para-medical professionals, who included a biochemist, translators and a photographer, Puharich and his colleagues, during a three weeks' stay, conducted intensive research, not only upon Arigó himself, but also into his diagnostic skill, treatment and progress in relation to a sample one thousand patients.

In each case Arigó explained in medical terms to the U.S. doctors his diagnosis of the particular patient. Puharich stressed that Arigó was very specific in his diagnoses, unhesitatingly designating, for example, the medical nature of a particular form of ulcer or defining types of blindness.

"In running 1,000 patients past him," said Puharich, "we found we were able to verify 550 verdicts, because in those cases we ourselves were able to establish a pretty definite diagnosis of what the problem was. In the remaining 450 cases, for example in rare blood cases, we could not be certain of our own diagnosis because we lacked available on-the-spot resources to enable us to do so. But of those of which we were certain we did not find a single case in which Arigó was at fault. This is fantastic!"

The doctors had questioned him. "How do you do this?" He had jovially replied: "It is the easiest thing in the world. A voice talks to me in my right ear and tells me the diagnosis." The voice, said Arigó, is that of Dr Fritz, said to be a German who died in 1918 in Estonia. Concerning this claim, Puharich reported that despite extensive inquiry—including a two-year library research —they had not been able to track down any records, but research continued in the light of new leads given by Arigó. When Puharich asked him: "How do you hear this voice?" he was told: "I hear it speaking in Portuguese—my own Portuguese."

Describing Arigó's diagnostic abilities as "absolutely pheno-menal", the doctor told us: "I would like to match him up against ten of the world's greatest medical diagnosticians. It would be very interesting to see how they would fare under similar conditions—just looking at people!"

Pointing out that many of Arigó's patients are in desperate plight who have come to Congonhas as a "Court of last appeal", Puharich said that data they had collected from patients regarded by doctors as "terminal cases" showed that about 5 per cent of them had been bluntly told the true state of affairs. In this section of the seemingly medically doomed, Arigó himself told about one in twenty: "Sorry, your time has come. I cannot do anything for you. God bless you." Another 10 per cent of patients in the severely ill category were given some alleviatory prescription. But with the remaining 85 per cent of so-called "incurable patients", "Arigó just goes ahead and treats."

As a result of the ever-intensifying pressure of patients who sought aid—the daily number was estimated to range upwards of 250 to as many as 1,000—Puharich reported that "timing tests" carried out over the years revealed that incredibly the healer had managed to halve his former average time of one minute per patient.

Puharich also confirmed the findings of other doctors who had studied Arigó, relating to the complexity of many prescriptions which might cover anything from four to as many as fifteen drugs. He said medical and registered trade names were always correctly given, and in the correct ratio, though the prescribed doses might often be much higher than normal.

Puharich said: "We never found a mistake in the name of a drug, the quantity sold or recommended dosage. He was phenomenally accurate in writing out his prescriptions, though he rarely bothered even to look at his writing." But even here the element of mystery was marked. Puharich confirmed that doctors who had tried out some of Arigó's prescriptions on other people with similar illnesses did not get equally striking results. He says: "Apparently the drugs themselves were not the sole answer. Something was at work which we just don't understand yet."

Arigó's surgical operations may justifiably be described as the unthinkable frequently triumphing over the impossible. Puharich laughingly likened it to "doing surgery in the middle of London's Victoria Station, in a rush hour, surrounded by mobs of children. It was unbelievable. It was chaos. It was just something that is almost impossible to believe but I tell it to you as I have seen it."

He gave a typical instance of a patient suffering from a disease of the small bowel, very difficult to treat and cure. Arigó told the man to drop his pants. Then he picked up a knife, wiped it on his shirt, slit the man open, pulled the patient's abdominal muscles apart, brought out the intestines and coolly chopped off a section as you would slice a sausage. Arigó then held the two ends of "dirty bowel", put them back and pulled the stomach walls together. Puharich confirmed that Arigó never used sutures. "And to cap all," said Puharich, "Arigó gave the chap a big punch in the belly and said 'that's it'."

Puharich also described Arigó's seemingly brusque but highly effective treatments of psychoses. He said that in the case of a young woman patient whom he considered to be a case of "severe schizophrenic background", but which Arigó described as "simply a matter of spirit possession", the healer had given her "three hard raps on her head. Remarkably enough it seemed to work." In the case of another woman whose EEG (encephelograph pattern) had revealed epilepsy, Arigó had said it was "possession". Her husband had told Arigó she had been fooling around with Macumba—a form of black magic. The doctor said: "She fell to the ground and went into what I thought was a typical Jacksonian epilepsy, but Arigó just slapped her so hard I thought he would fracture her jaw. She has never had any similar attack since."

Commenting on Arigó's famous "eye check-ups"—also shown in a film taken by his team—Puharich confirmed what I myself had witnessed and experienced when I had placed a finger on the patient's eyebrow and felt the knife blade dug deep into the gristly eyebrow tissue. Puharich had also been asked by Arigó to take hold of the knife blade in this position. He told me after the lecture: "It is a strange thing because although the blade was dug deep into the man's eye there appeared to be no fluidity of tissue in the interior, almost as if the blade were driving between the cells." A brave man, Puharich had asked Arigó to perform the same "check-up" on him, but Arigó did not do so.

Confirming that Arigó had on occasion been offered fantastic sums for his services, he told us: "To my knowledge he never accepted a penny for his work, yet over the years I have seen as many as one thousand patients treated in a day—the equivalent of those seen at the large New York hospital where I work. His work load was truly enormous."

Describing the results of extensive electro-cardiac, biochemical, physiological and psychological tests carried out on Arigó during the team's visit to Brazil in May 1968 and January 1969, Puharich said: "The net result was that Arigó was found to be perfectly normal. Furthermore, in all the time we have studied him we never found the slightest hint of fraud, sleight of hand or chicanery."

Now six Brazilian doctors had been persuaded to sponsor a research clinic at Congonhas. This would not only provide a medical umbrella of protection for Arigó's healing activities but also provide needed research facilities for all visiting researchers.

Summing up the challenge presented to medical researchers by Arigó's many-faceted achievements, Dr Puharich said frankly: "In regard to Arigó's own statement that he was simply a 'tool or instrument manipulated by the spirit personality of Dr Fritz', our scientific skills were unfortunately so limited we have no way of proving such a personality existed. We can only say he *did* these things and that he had medical genius, either his own, or genius at one step removed. At the moment I am open-minded, and I suspect we shall be working on these problems for many years to come. He does it. I can't tell you how. He certainly provides one of the most fruitful sources of knowledge, information and opportunity for sincere, skilled, dedicated scientists to study, for his one-man output per week is equivalent to that of a fairly large hospital, and I suspect its batting average is just as good. At the moment I find him probably one of the most remarkable objects of study I have ever encountered, and we are preparing our material in the hope that some medical journal will accept our evidence."

13. Spirit Hospitals

Among the many hundreds of charitable foundations established by Brazilian Spiritists none presents a greater challenge to Western orthodoxy, particularly medicine, than the "Sanatorios Espiritas", or Spirit hospitals for the mentally ill. Sometimes picturesquely described as hospitals for the healing of "illnesses of the soul", they deserve to be more widely known and studied. The work now being carried out within their confines by teams of unpaid administrators and healers may well herald the dawn of a revolutionized approach to the growing world scourge of mental illness which afflicts all societies, not least the affluent nations and the culturally proud.

Ironically, in a century technologically triumphant, when it is men's boast that even outer space is becoming increasingly submissive to their probing craft, soaring graphs of mind sickness silently mock man's empirical conquests.

Even in Britain's vaunted welfare state it is a sad fact that one woman in every nine and one man in every fourteen are likely to need hospital treatment for mental illness at some time in their lives. Indeed, mental patients occupy nearly half of all available hospital beds in the country, claiming a victim from one in every five families.

The size and complexity of the problem facing modern medicine is well exemplified in schizophrenia, commonest, and one of the most tragic, forms of insanity which appears to be on the increase. Its causes still baffle medical experts, yet it has been estimated that over 20 per cent of all new admissions into mental hospitals come within this category and that over 50 per cent of those remaining in hospital will be sufferers from one or other of the schizophrenic psychoses. Worse, it is the persecutor of youth, for some two-thirds of the victims are claimed between the ages of 15 and 30—hence the term *dementia praecox* (early dementia) which was the official designation before the term schizophrenia became preferred.

Against this backcloth, the medical challenge presented by Brazil's spirit hospitals is primarily reflected in the fact that orthodox medical treatments—such as electric shock, insulin comas and tranquillizing drugs—administered by paid qualified medical staff, are supplemented with daily sessions of spiritual healing given by visiting teams of unpaid healer-mediums.

During my Brazilian visit I was privileged to visit four such hospitals, including the largest, oldest and best known, situated in Porto Alegre, capital of Brazil's southernmost state, Rio Grande do Sul. This 42-year-old hospital, with the recent completion of a fine new seven-storey wing, now boasts 600 beds.

It is a fascinating paradox that over the past century the remarkable growth of Spiritism in Brazil, a land which has often been described as "the brightest jewel in the Roman Catholic diadem", has been closely linked with the work of outstanding medical men, particularly homoeopathic doctors favouring a combination of medical and spiritual therapies.

Hahnemann, founder of homoeopathic medicine, was one of the first to recognize that many diseases are psychosomatic in origin, though his fame primarily rests upon his inoculation-type treatment of disease by minute doses of drugs that in a healthy person produce symptoms similar to the disease.

Although his theories have always been strongly challenged, Hahnemann, who died in 1843, was undoubtedly far ahead of his time in realizing that physical illness was all too frequently only the outward symptom of inner psychic and spiritual disease. In his introduction to *Organon* he stated: "Diseases will not cease to be spiritual dynamic derangements of our spiritual vital principle."

He believed that it was of vital importance, when seeking to cure physical ills by medical means, simultaneously to enlist the aid of spiritual therapy aimed at making "the soul react in search of a cure." This heretical, dualistic approach to illness had a cogent appeal for Brazilians who temperamentally may be said to possess a national genius for combining mysticism and magic.

The historical accident of a friendly correspondence between Hahnemann and José Bonifacio de Andrada, a Brazilian statesman who later became revered as the "Patriarch" of his country's battle for independence from the chains of Portuguese colonialism, proved fateful.

José Bonifacio was a prominent member of one of the first groups of neo-Spiritualists in the Western world. And the fruitful consequences of his friendship with Hahnemann undoubtedly helped to shape the subsequent unique pattern and growth of Brazilian Spiritism in the ensuing century. Indeed, Pedro McGregor goes so far as to state that it was, in fact, through homoeopathic medicine that Spiritism was able to penetrate so successfully in the Roman Catholic citadel of Brazil.

Certainly the views of these two disparately gifted men, particularly those of Hahnemann, strongly influenced the work of two doctors: a Portuguese, Joao Vicente Martins and a Frenchman, Dr Mure, who practised in Brazil in the 1840s. McGregor tells us that these two men, who devoted their major professional efforts to treating the poor free of charge, supplemented their homoeopathic medicine with "magnetic treatment". This consisted of passing their outstretched hands over the patient at a distance of three to four inches, as they prayed for God's help in the cure.

Hahnemann, himself, had privately recommended the use of the healing "pass" as an auxiliary aid to effecting cures. Such healing passes, of course, remain a basic feature of Spiritual healing today in many countries.

And as the cornerstone of its astonishing success, Brazilian Spiritism also eventually adopted a slogan originally coined by Martins and Mure: God, Christ and Charity.

During this period of the nineteenth-century another medical doctor, later destined to become President of Brazil's State Assembly in 1880, was growing up. Widely admired for his courage, talents and idealism, Dr Adolfo Bezerra de Menezes, who has been dubbed the "Paul" of Brazilian Spiritism, also became President of the Brazilian Spiritist Federation.

Of his own chosen profession he wrote:

A true doctor does not have the right to finish his meal, to choose the time, to ask whether the call comes from near or far, on the hill or in the suburbs. The man who does not answer because he has visitors, because it is late at night or because a client cannot pay, is not a doctor but a dealer in medicine, someone who works to collect interest on the capital invested in his schooling.

Appalled both by the social neglect in his day of the mentally ill, and the medical ignorance concerning the causes of such illnesses he was the first man in Brazil publicly to advocate a controversial alliance between spiritual and medical therapies in this field. He strongly held the view that the statement of the Nazarene that men could cure lunatics by casting out "the demons that possessed them", was no mere figure of speech.

As we shall see, many years later the views of this good doctor were courageously translated into practice by the seven dedicated founders of Brazil's first Spiritist hospital in Porto Alegre.

Meanwhile Menezes, like many other of his colleagues, was decisively influenced by the theories of another famous nineteenth-century Frenchman, Léon Denizarth Hippolyte Rivail, better known to millions of readers today of his best-selling book *The Spirits' Book*—bible of Brazilian Spiritism—under his pen-name "Allan Kardec".

Rivail, like Hahnemann and Menezes, was another pioneer bridge-builder who refused to accept the increasing schism separating men of science and men of religion. He believed the time had come for the teaching of Christ to be complemented by science. In his book *Genesis* he affirmed : "Science and religion are two levers of human intelligence : one reveals the law of the material world and the other of the moral world. But, both having the same principle—God—they cannot contradict one another."

Born in Lyons, but educated in Protestant Switzerland, Rivail, a successful schoolmaster and author of many educational text-books still used in French schools, became an ardent psychic researcher. At heart a religious reformer who cherished a deep desire to create a greater degree of unity between the various Christian sects, he embarked upon a protracted experiment with two young amateur mediums, daughters of a friend. Through their mediumship, expressed in table-rapping and planchette-writing, he sought answers to a series of linked questions relating to fundamental problems of human life and the universe.

When these two-world communications had been going on twice a week for nearly two years he confessed to his wife : "It is a curious thing, my conversations with the invisible intelligences have completely revolutionized my ideas and convictions."

His first issue of *The Spirits' Book* brought immediate success and Rivail founded the Parisian Society of Psychological Studies for the purpose of obtaining further information through a much wider circle of mediums. Weekly meetings were held in his home.

Similar associations were formed in other countries and eventually, from an extraordinary mass of spirit-teachings called from an ever-widening variety of sources over a period of 15 years, Kardec collated, co-ordinated and cross-checked an enlarged, revised edition. Published in 1857 it is this edition which became the recognized text-book of the school of Spiritualist philosophy which today counts its "Spiritist" followers in millions, particularly in Brazil.

The word "Spiritist" was coined by Kardec. He wrote :

Strictly speaking, everyone is a Spiritualist who believes that there is in him something more than matter, but it does not follow that he believes in the existence of spirits, or in their communication with the visible world. Instead, therefore, of the words Spiritual, Spiritualism, we employ to designate this latter belief by the words Spiritist, Spiritism, which by their form indicate their origin and radical meaing. We say then, that the fundamental principle of the Spiritist theory, or Spiritism, is the relation of the material world with spirits, or the beings of the invisible world : and we designate the adherents of the Spiritist theory as Spiritists.

A convinced believer in reincarnation as a necessary road to eventual perfection, Rivail summed up the "moral teaching of the higher spirits" in the words of Christ : "Do unto others as you would that others should do unto you."

Four years after Rivail's death at his desk on March 31, 1869, a Brazilian group predominantly consisting of homoeopathic doctors was founded under the name "Group Confucius". They published the first Portuguese translation of Kardec's main works: *The Spirits' Book, The Book of Mediums,* and the *Gospels According to Spiritism.* Their sales are estimated to have exceeded a million-and-a-half copies. Members of the Confucius Group, inspired, like their forerunners, by a spirit of compassion and service, adopted the "Kardec" slogan: "Without Charity there is no Salvation."

McGregor, himself a gifted spiritual healer, in his historical analysis of Brazilian Spiritism,* tells us:

"Charity, indeed, was to become the driving force behind Spiritism in Brazil. It took two main forms: spiritual healing and social assistance to the poor. . . . The spiritual healing practised in Brazil took on an entirely different form to that known in England and the United States of America. In the first place, Brazilian mediums actually receive medical prescriptions which are dictated to them through a spirit guide. The medium is known as a healing-medium and the prescriptions are mostly homoeopathic. The *Group Confucius* was the first to establish an organization dispensing a free service of homoeopathic prescriptions given through healing-mediums on certain days of the week.

"Secondly, and perhaps more important, mediumship was exercised under the evangelical motto *Give freely what you have received freely* (Matthew 10.8, 'Heal the sick, cleanse the lepers, raise the dead, cast out devils: freely ye have received, freely give . . .').

"Here were no entrance fees, subscriptions, silver collections or requests for financial help to defray costs. The majority of the practitioners were well-to-do professional people and the prescriptions really were fulfilled without any charge whatever.

"These two factors, total and genuine lack of cost to the healed and treatment by specific medicaments 'prescribed' by spirits rather than generalized healing through their aid, are the main differences between Brazilian and other branches of the movement."

He also assures us that the chief "spirit doctors" signing the prescriptions delivered through healing-mediums were believed to be none other than Doctors Bento Mure and Joao Vicente Martins, the two men who had first introduced homoeopathy to Brazil.

Certainly as a pace-setter Brazilian Spiritism is unbeatable.

* *The Moon and Two Mountains* by Pedro McGregor.

Today the original free homoeopathic service founded by the Group Confucius has burgeoned into over 1700 social assistance establishments throughout the sub-continent. Even within the past two decades—on estimates backed both by official statistics and the dismayed numerical accounting of Roman Catholic authorities—the number of Brazilian Spiritists has increased tenfold from 1 million at the 1950 census to a present estimated 10 million.

Official statistics also testify that while Roman Catholics numerically represent more than 90 percent of the country's population, Catholic social assistance establishments comprise only 42 per cent of the total, yet Spiritists, officially listed as only 1.5 per cent of the population, contribute no less than 36 per cent of all such establishments. In the state of São Paulo alone, economically and industrially the most advanced in Brazil, Spiritist schools in the nine years from 1950 to 1958 increased from 9 to 43; hospitals from 1 to 13; shelters and orphanages from 11 to 47 and libraries from 59 to over 100.

FIRST SPIRIT HOSPITAL

Resembling at night a giant jewelled starfish in concrete, sprawled over the incline of a low hill on the southern outskirts of the city, Porto Alegre's Spirit Hospital represents the impressive fulfilment of an impossible dream born in 1912—a dream shared by seven men of widely varying talents.

Members of an Allan Kardec Spiritist Society, these visionary initiators of Brazil's breakthrough in the field of mental therapy had become deeply distressed over the plight of psychopaths and the mentally ill in Brazil. Even as late as 1912 they were all too frequently condemned to a life-sentence of confinement with little or no hope of cure.

Deeply impressed by the theories of Dr Adolfo Bezerra de Menezes expressed in his treatise *Insanity from a Different Perspective*, they finally decided to put his ideas to the test.

The combined professional and practical experience of the seven men proved admirably effective for such a venture, for the group of friends comprised two medical doctors, two civil engineers, a Senator, a civil servant and an author-professor. After fourteen years of patient, arduous effort the dream eventually took shape in the modest form of a 36-bed hospital, officially opened on Christmas Day, 1926, in the Avenida Cel. Lucas de Oliveira.

It was a proud moment for the seven hospital directors, especially for Dr Oscar Pitthan, medical founder and principal instigator in 1912 of the non-profit-making society which they had formed to back the unique project.

Dr Pitthan's six colleagues were: Dr Henrique Inacio Domingues, a fellow-physician; Dr Augusto Pestana, a well-known civil engineer, ex-Federal Deputy and a former director of the State Railways; Dr A. Verissimo de Mattos, civil engineer and a former director of the State's River Board; Col. Frederico A. Gomes da Silva, a leading official in the State's Finance Department; Algemiro Morem, a merchant, and Professor Alfonso Guerreiro Lima, author.

Generous help and encouragement was also given by Dona Maria de la Granje Mostadeiro. She not only made a gift of land and a considerable financial contribution towards the building of the first hospital, but also later became its first resident President. In 1934 the hospital had become so firmly established that the need to expand became correspondingly urgent. A larger piece of land was purchased in the suburb of Teresopolis, site of the present repeatedly enlarged building.

Building of the first wing of the present building on this site, which commands superb views of the Guaiba estuary, was started in 1940 and opened on February 2 of the following year.

The second wing was inaugurated on September 7, 1951. The third wing has now provided not only an additional 230 beds but also new workshops, service departments and improved administrative facilities, including a modern laundry.

The hospital's visiting book contains many enthusiastic tributes, including the following testimony from Dr Adauto Botelho, a leading psychiatrist and General Director of the National Department for Assistance to the Insane, who visited the hospital on May 20, 1944. His official tribute might well be said to mark the "coming of age" of the hospital's acceptance by an important section of the medical profession.

Dr Botelho wrote: "I have visited, with great pleasure and

professional satisfaction, this spirit hospital about which I cannot conceal my praise of the medical work that is being done therein, as well as the humanitarian treatment to which it is dedicated.

"May the hospital at all times continue on these lines so that its directors may always merit the eulogies which they so justly deserve, practising the Profession of medicine in accordance with its highest precepts and exercising that charity which emanates from the heart and from true altruism."

Senhor Conrado Ferrari, septuagenarian President of the Porto Alegre Spirit Hospital, who made me warmly welcome, is unquestionably one of the busiest "retired" men in Brazil. Formerly the administrative chief of the State's Federal University in Porto Alegre, both he and his devoted wife, Ida, give so much of their time to the hospital that they not only spend most of their days in it but many nights too.

In February, 1969 Senhor Ferrari told me in a letter: "Our hospital continues to progress with a daily average of 500 hospitalized patients. The two buildings that were being started when you were here are now finished, providing our hospital with a total capacity of 600 beds and extended services. A further wing is now being constructed to provide additional medical offices, dental and administrative services."

The ever-increasing medical respect shown for the work done in this hospital is reflected in the fact that 15 psychiatrists send their own patients to the hospital for treatment.

Senhor Ferrari told me that since the hospital does not receive a formal state subsidy, other than exemption from taxes as a registered charity and, in the past, an occasional subsidy from the government, the administrators have had to increase the provision for paying patients who now provide 75 per cent of the hospital's income, the remainder being raised by individual donations, a welcome proportion of these coming from doctors.

But admittance of paying patients to meet soaring inflationary costs, is *not* reflected in any special privileges for the more wealthy patients. Certainly the new wing includes additional bathroom suites, some of them also including a small sitting room, but in regard to all other aspects—medical treatment, food and available communal amenities—there is no distinction made between paying and non-paying patients. And Senhora Ferrari's days are largely occupied in running an extensive department, staffed by volunteer workers, to provide hospital and other clothing for needy patients.

The aims and principles of the hospital also remain unchanged :

1. The spirit hospital is the fruit of the idealism and endeavour of Rio Grande do Sul Spiritists. Its purpose is not to make profits but to shelter and to treat those who are spiritually unwell, giving them of the best at the lowest cost to themselves, welcoming and treating without payment those who cannot afford to contribute, with the same tender care.
2. The personnel responsible for the maintenance of the establishment have no rights, but merely duties, and the directors are not paid for their services.
3. Neuro-psychiatric patients are received without any distinction as to religion, race or social position. All are given the same food and treatment, whether they be contributors or otherwise.
4. The Institution has its own medical staff but its doors are always open to specialists, duly authorized by the competent official department, wishing to hospitalize and attend their own patients therein.

Naturally my short stay in Porto Alegre which included visits on two successive days to the hospital provided inadequate opportunity for me to attempt to convey any analysis of its scope and significance. Neither am I qualified, as a mere laywoman, to comment upon the efficacy or otherwise of the therapies practised within its walls. I can only tell you that the hospital facilities and amenities provided in this fine building—the treatment and patients' wards, recreation, psychotherapy facilities and dining halls—impressed me favourably as bearing comparison with those I have seen over the years in two large mental hospitals I have had occasion to visit, one of them situated in the North of England, and the other in Outer London.

On the day I lunched in Porto Alegre with members of the administrative staff in one of the hospital's spacious white and red-tiled dining halls, the spotless, well equipped kitchens catered for a total of 239 resident patients and 115 hospital staff.

Our luncheon that day, as served to the patients also, consisted of a nourishing and palatable soup, a french beans and tomato salad, tasty meat stew served with well cooked rice and the traditional Brazilian beans, a sweet from the tropical fruit mamao, and coffee.

During my tour of the hospital I garnered a mountain of statistics, ranging from patients' records to monthly hospital expenditure on psychiatric drugs—including glucose supplies, insulin injections and neozine. But statistics alone, though apparently impressive in the case of this hospital, do not in themselves reflect the underlying importance of the work carried out in spirit hospitals.

Rather does this lie in two linked fields. The first I can best describe as a strong personal impression I gained in the four hospitals I visited, of an exceptional friendly warmth at every level—a feeling almost of a family-concern relationship linking patients and staff.

The second lies in the nature of the varied "psychic" and medical therapies used and the spiritual perspectives opened up by the achievements in this field—perspectives which would appear to challenge not only the present bounds of medical and psychiatric attitudes but also those of orthodox religion and exclusively materialist-based science.

During my visit to Porto Alegre I was privileged, with the help of my young translator, to have several long and frank conversations with the hospital president, Senhor Conrado Ferrari, a remarkable man I came both to like and respect profoundly.

Formerly a public functionary widely esteemed in varying responsible capacities—Senhor Ferrari was a former Prefect of his native city—he has simultaneously also acted as unpaid President of the hospital since 1933, and edits the hospital's widely circulated monthly journal "Desobsessao".

At the time of my visit the family links with the hospital's progress not only included Senhor Ferrari's wife, Ida, but also their son who is one of four full-time doctors employed at the hospital. Both Senhor Ferrari and his wife are modest about their own personal contribution to the hospital's astonishing success, emphasizing that this rests upon the firm foundation of team co-operation at every level combined with broad-based tolerance and acceptance of varying viewpoints and specializations.

And undoubtedly the best tribute to the work of the pioneering hospital can be found in the following frank answers given by Senhor Ferrari—and other doctors and psychiatrists associated directly and indirectly with the hospital—to a questionnaire I submitted for answers and translation.

Here are Senhor Ferrari's answers to questions I put to him.

Q. 1.   *Are all kinds of mental illness treated, for example, paranoia, schizophrenia, etc.?*

Answer : In this hospital we treat all types of mental and nervous diseases, including alcoholism and drug addiction. Regarding procedure, when a patient is admitted he is first interviewed by a psychiatrist on the day of arrival and the latter makes an initial diagnosis in his written report. The patient is also given a medical examination by the doctor in charge of the clinics and an electro-cardiogram analysis. The doctor recommends suitable treatment, for example, electric shock treatment or insulin coma. An ophthalmologist carries out eye examinations and the hospital laboratory carries out all necessary tests requested by the doctor. Medical treatment commences immediately. Another psychiatrist carries out a second interview and submits a separate report, confirming or otherwise, the initial diagnosis.

Similar interviews and examinations are carried out periodically during the patient's stay in the hospital and full records of medical and psychiatric treatment are preserved in the hospital's files as well as details of daily treatment and drugs.

Simultaneously, and with the consent of the patient and relatives, healing passes are daily given by healing-mediums. There is a team of visiting mediums for every day of the week. In cases where obsession is indicated, absent healing is administered—i.e. the patient is not present—at evening seances organized twice weekly by the administration within the hospital. Absent healing is also given at separate sessions, when requested, to patients outside the hospital, sometimes in neighbouring countries, for example, Argentina. Distance presents no difficulty. For absent healing experiments we only require the name and address of the patient.

Q. 2.   *Is mental illness increasing in Brazil? If so, why?*

Answer: In Brazil, as in the rest of the world, mental illness is increasing. Doctors say this is due to present emotional pressures such as the possibility of total war, following two world wars and world-wide economic problems. Sexual problems, alcoholism and drug addiction are other major factors.

Spiritists, however, believe the primary cause arises from the fact that we are at present living in a difficult period of transition prior to a new era which will offer happier prospects for those who survive the impending holocaust. In other words we are suffering the birth-pangs which precede every New Age for I believe we are living in the Apocalyptic period predicted by St John.

Q. 3.   *How do doctors regard "obsession" cases?*

Answer: Though some doctors accept the phenomenon of obsession, professionally they prefer to ignore it for we believe they are afraid of criticism from their medical Association which here, as in other parts of the world, holds orthodox views. The doctors who work at our hospital are not Spiritualists so we could not get their views on obsession. Such obsessional phenomena as clairvoyance, hearing voices and so on are regarded by them as mere "hallucinations".

The practice of black magic, a grave problem in Brazil, is definitely a factor in obsession cases. Revenge is another prevalent Karmic cause. We treat some terrible cases of really conscienceless "obsessing" entities but after we explain through a medium the consequences to themselves if they continue to persecute their living victims we can make them become afraid. When this happens more evolved spirits can take them in hand and arrange treatment in Spirit hospitals on the other side.

In obsession treatments the difference in the patient can be seen by the following day. As Spiritists we are convinced that our high percentage of successful treatments at this hospital is due to this work, though the doctors, of course, naturally attribute such cures to their own medical treatments. We are content to leave it at that.

Q. 4. *Is your percentage of relapses higher or lower than the norm for Brazil?*

Answer : We do not have statistics on relapses. From the psychiatric standpoint every "schizophrenic" is subject to periodic returns to the hospital. Remissions in these cases are rare. As Spiritists we regard many of the patients classified by doctors as "schizophrenic" as being "obsessional" cases. These are treated mediumistically by removing the obsessors as I have already described. It must be said, however, that if the patient does not then play *his* part in consolidating the healing carried out, i.e. by developing his psychic powers if he is a budding medium, or by mending his ways if the obsession has been caused by bad habits, or learning to forgive his enemies, then he may again relapse, for the healing of obsession depends ultimately *more* upon the patient himself than those who seek to help him. We only carry out emergency treatment.

Q. 5. *Are Spiritist hospitals greatly at a disadvantage compared with orthodox mental hospitals in regard to State subsidies?*

Answer : Our hospital has received governmental subsidies, but not regularly. It has primarily depended on the men who are in government, though we believe there is no actual ban against us for being a Spiritist institution. Of course it is natural that in Brazil, where the majority of the population declare themselves Catholic, the hospitals headed by priests and nuns should receive larger subsidies than we do.

Q. 6. *Can you give instances of persecution of extreme prejudice a) from doctors b) the state c) the Roman Catholic Church, past or present?*

Answer : We have not been subject to persecution against the hospital by any of the above-named, although doctors were prejudiced about a Spiritist organization actually building a hospital, and priests have warned their followers against the heresy of Spiritism.

Today the Spirit hospital in Porto Alegre is respected

by all types of Brazilian medical insitutions, because of
its progress and improved technical and nursing conditions, though there remains a certain dislike of the name
"Spirit". Many doctors have urged the need to change
this name as a means of securing better support from the
medical profession. We have not done so because we
have gained the respect of the public, as well as respect
in medical and governmental circles, despite the title
and we do not want to pander to unjust prejudice.

Q. 7. *Can present teamwork between mediums and doctors
in Spirit hospitals be improved?*

Answer : We would like to emulate the example set by Dr Inacio
Ferreira, head of the Uberaba Spirit Hospital. He is
a doctor *and* a Spiritist. Young people are being prepared for such work for we try to enlist their interest and
give them the opportunity to work as interns in our
hospital. We certainly hope at some future date to have
a medical team who could accept medical *and* mediumistic therapeutics, both being applied by doctors. This
won't be easy to achieve since the materialist and orthodox views at present held in Universities and Medical
Associations present obstacles and make doctors reluctant openly to declare themselves Spiritists. Meanwhile there are encouraging signs. Our hospital is now a
big organization and the only mental hospital in this
state that receives patients coming from other doctors.
The other hospitals only accept patients who are
treated by their own doctors. This situation inevitably
causes an encouraging number of doctors to be associated with our organization.

Q. 8. *Do you think that Spirit hospitals have a permanent
place in a) Brazilian medicine b) world medicine?*

Answer : Pubic opinion has changed very much in relation to this
hospital. In the early years there was a certain prejudice
which caused many people to look askance at becoming
resident patients. But with the passing of time and
because of the good treatment patients receive in the
hospital, the situation has improved. Today there are
many who *prefer* the treatment received in this hospital
and indeed a considerable number seek us out just
because of our healer-mediums. To sum up I would

say that prejudice is exceptional, mainly confined to people who don't think for themselves.

I also think the hospital has won a definite place not only in Brazil but also in the world of medicine. We employ medical methods that bear comparison with those employed in any civilized country. As Spiritists we also carry out spiritual therapies, but in doing so we endeavour not to create any difficulties for the doctors, so there is perfect harmony. Our doctors do not interfere in the mediumistic service, and the mediums don't interfere in the medical area.

Q. 9.   *Would you welcome visiting research teams of doctors, psychiatrists, psychic researchers, etc. from other countries?*

Answer :   For our part, as Spiritists, medical teams or researchers coming from other countries would be welcomed, to study and observe the methods used in our hospital. I cannot answer for our Head Doctor who is responsible to the relevant Government Ministry for the hospital's performance.

In regard to our work on "obsession cases" we have attended emergency cases coming from Argentina and other countries, including the United States. We have done what we could and according to information received later the effects were beneficial.

Within three months of my return to England from Brazil in 1967 Senhor Ferrari very kindly sent to me the views of four leading psychiatrists in the state of Rio Grande do Sul who had studied copies of the questionnaire I had formulated. All gave permission for publication of their views.

The men concerned are Dr Ivo Castilhos Puignau, a specialist in psychosomatic illnesses; Dr Nelson Aspesi, neurologist, Assistant of the Chair of Neurology at the School of Medicine at the Federal University of Rio Grande do Sul (Dr Aspesi is also President of the State's "Psychiatric, Neurologist and Neuro-Surgery Society"); Dr José Theobaldo Diefenthaeler, described by Senhor Ferrari as : "One of the leading psychiatrists in Porto Alegre. Not a Spiritist"; and Dr Nelson Lemos, described as a psychiatrist of the orthodox school.

All the above had been treating their own patients at the Porto Alegre hospital over periods ranging from five to eight years.

All answered "Yes" to my question: "Has the spirit hospital given you the necessary facilities, conditions, nursing and collaboration to enable you to treat patients admitted into the hospital?"

Dr Puignau described the spirit hospital as "the best hospital in the city and one of the best in Brazil, offering good conditions for work not only in respect to the atmosphere but also as regards the nursing staff."

Dr Jose Theobaldo Diefenthaeler described it as "an excellent psychiatric hospital within its condition of a 'monoblock house' and large hospital."

In answer to a follow-up question: "How does it compare with similar Brazilian institutions?" Dr Puignau replied: "It can be compared with the best ones." Dr Aspesi said: "I have no opinion." Dr Diefenthaeler said he had incorporated his answer in the foregoing reply quoted, while Dr Nelson Lemos stated: "Yes. It depends on the patient's relatives' criteria. It is valuable according to the faith of relatives and patients."

Regarding spiritual assistance given to many patients by visiting teams of mediums all four doctors said they were aware of this and did not object since it was not "imposed" by the hospital as a condition of hospitalization.

Dr Puignau commented: "I not only know, but I constantly request spiritual assistance for those patients who need it." In regard to cases of "obsession" he declared: "In some cases, after passing through the hands of well-known colleagues I have observed that the cases were of 'obsession', or, as they would say, to use the words of the Gospel, 'possessed', 'mad' and that [they] were healed by mediumistic development and by the treatment of the patient himself."

Dr Aspesi stated he did not have "enough facts scientifically to say whether it is useful or not".

Dr Lemos described spiritual treatment as: "Useful or harmful, depending on the relatives' disposition to accept or reject the assistance, and the same applies to patients."

Asked to comment on whether there was a favourable or unfavourable difference in the percentage of cures and positive improvements in patients, as between the Spirit hospital and other mental hospitals, three of the psychiatrists said they had not enough data to pass an opinion. Two of these added the comment that they believed the results were similar.

Dr Puignau wrote: "The percentage of healings or improvements (for the Spiritist hospital) is larger than in other similar institutions."

Asked if they would care to present a critique as to the methods followed in Spirit hospitals the psychiatrists answered as follows:

Dr Puignau: "Methods depend on the doctor. The spirit hospital presents good facilities, though it does not have everything that is necessary, for the building is not yet finished [the new wing has since come into operation. Author.] I think time will change for the better everything that exists.

"As to the methods employed by myself, they are different in each case, using the therapeutics described in the Gospel and the resources of the Reincarnation Law as well as the 'deobsession' processes. There are many other resources but I do not use them. It is clear that psychotherapy and hypnosis are very valuable in the cure of unbalanced human beings."

Dr Puignau added the following comments: "I believe that the patients can be divided into two groups: those who are psychically injured, for whom nothing else can be done, and those who are partially injured or are heading for injuries. The latter group could be greatly helped by medical science if the problems of madness could be seen from a new viewpoint, say that of Dr Bezerra de Menezes, a marvellous Brazilian who opened up new horizons in spiritual therapy.

"However, the sick man and child are considered in an isolated context, and never as they have lived. In their former lives are to be found the real causes of the major infirmities, also of their spiritual enemies.

"The 'Fathers' of modern psychiatry, not realizing these facts or understanding mediumistic phenomena, could only do as they have done.

"It is necessary to open up vistas in the direction of the spiritual. Only atheists have the right to ignore the Gospel and biblical facts, from Nebuchadnezzar to Babylon. Christians must research into the prophetic dreams (clairvoyance?) of Joseph in Egypt to supernormal phenomena in the Gospels. Do not the latter speak of the 'spirit' descended upon the crowd when thousands started to speak in different languages? An atheist would say 'madness', but why not take a fresh look at all existing theories. Not to do so is to be unscientific."

Dr Aspesi wrote : "As a neurologist I have had opportunity to use all my knowledge, but I would like, if possible, to see more opportunities for secondary examinations." He concludes his answers with the comment : "In life and in medicine, love and security are backgrounds of basic value which should always be well cemented."

Similarly Dr Diefenthaeler contented himself with stating : "I would only like to emphasize that mental patients are only human beings, needing above all, help, love, comfort, and understanding."

Dr Lemos said he would like to see : "More emphasis placed on ambient-therapy with attendants skilled in talking to the patients and able to win a response."

A MEDICAL PROPHET?

And in this highly controversial field Brazil has found an eloquent advocate. Since it is the voice of a medically qualified "phophet", it cannot long go totally ignored, for Doctor Inacio Ferreira, author of *New Ways of Medicine* (two volumes) and *Psychiatry Face to Face with Reincarnation*, is well qualified to make his challenge. His fourteen years' medical training is backed with thirty-five years of psychiatric field experience in the treatment of mental illness.

This gentle-voiced, grey-haired, scholar-psychiatrist, who has his own modest country town practice as a specialist in nervous diseases, has at considerable cost to his own health and personal pocket, been for many years the unpaid medical director of Uberaba's small forty-bed spirit hospital.

I was told that in the past fourteen years he had never had a holiday away from the town where he attends the hospital daily. Now, urgent health considerations have forced him to take Saturdays off. He generally spends them in a little cottage in the nearby countryside.

When I visited him in this remote town five hours' flying distance from Rio in mid-west Brazil, he told me of the prejudice he had to surmount when he began his association with the hospital. "No doctors wanted to work in them," he told me, "because Spiritists faced much ignorant persecution. I myself wasn't keen at the commencement, but I became increasingly impressed." He has also publicly stated : "In the past I laughed at the idea of mediums with no medical training and some of them with little education of any kind, being able to heal cases that we doctors could not. Now, after studying this subject thoroughly, I bow before these untutored healers, for I have become convinced that such people can benefit 80 per cent of the mental illness that medicine fails to understand and refuses to study in a wider context."

He qualified this viewpoint by stressing that when the cause of mental illness is spiritual it is *not* schizophrenic. Emphasizing that it needs much experience and knowledge to be able to distinguish the spiritual from the material in mental illness, he told me : "In cases of true schizophrenia only 5 per cent get cured because medicine doesn't know the cause of this illness."

In the rural districts of the vast plain which surrounds Uberaba there is much poverty, and since the kindliness of this dedicated doctor is widely known he is sent tragic cases of the homeless and the ill picked up in desperate states by the police. Since at the time I visited him, Dr Ferreira had no other medical help and was primarily interested in patients who could be helped by a combination of medical and spiritual therapies (he can call upon the services of 20-30 visiting mediums who visit the hospital in daily groups) he was providing temporary shelter to such cases. When necessary he arranges their eventual transfers to orthodox hospitals.

He told me it was only within the past five years that he had been forced to ask any hospitalized patient for any payment. He said sadly : "Now I have to take some paying patients into the hospital though I still manage to accommodate one-third of the total free of any charge, the remainder paying what they can afford."

In contrast to such outstandingly well-equipped Spirit hospitals as the one I have described in Porto Alegre, Dr Ferreira's "Sanatorio Espirita de Uberaba" was pitifully ill-equipped. Although some of the accommodation I was shown which housed the more violent inmates was disturbingly primitive, there was eloquent evidence from the patients of a reciprocal affection and trust. Wherever we went they flocked round this tired benign man like children beseiging a loved father.

In the modest-sized, paint-peeling bungalow which is his home a short distance away from the hospital, the library is its chief glory, and much loved cats the princelings. Every moment he can wrest from his onerous professional responsibilities is spent at his desk where he has embarked on the third volume of his controversial contribution to medical literature.

Dr Ferreira believes that mental illnesses are frequently Karmic in origin, particularly cases of obsession. In his books he backs this view with an array of startling case histories. I cannot comment on their medical soundness, nor does my scant knowledge of the riddles of reincarnation enable me to pass any judgement for or against the theory. All I can tell you is that the handful of cases I have been privileged to read in translations present formidable social and philosophic implications, for they seem to indicate that we cannot hope effectively to cope even with the psychiatric problems of alcoholism or crimes of violence, unless we begin to take at least a closer look at the seemingly fantastic possibility that—in Dr Ferreira's words—"Reincarnation provides the key."

He stresses: "The basis of all life is the psychic life. In order that medicine should really fulfil its mission it must extend the battle to psychic *causes*. It must study the laws of spiritual immortality and reincarnation." He also warns that since in many cases psychic and organic illnesses are indissolubly linked there is increasingly a need to "ally psychic treatment to organic treatment". In this view he certainly is *not* alone.

Of alcoholism he writes: "It makes a hell of everyone's life associated with the victim but science cannot give direct help because it has not found the cause *behind* alcoholism. Materialism! Materialism! They overlook *psychic* heredity with all its vices and intoxication of the spirit. They blame present environment and bad friends in this life, but the real causes lie deeper. They do not realize they can even be imbedded in the past. They do not realize that psychic injuries from the past can reflect in pathological tendencies and effects."

Like his friend Senhor Conrado Ferrari, Dr Ferreira is in possession of many tragic case histories which he, too, believes point to Other Side vendettas carried out against the living by obsessing "entities" in revenge for injuries said to have been inflicted in past incarnations.

Both men would welcome visits by open-minded medical men and scientific researchers, particularly from England and the United States, to study the work now being carried out in Spirit hospitals, frequently under appalling difficulties. To this I add my own insignificant plea, for no matter how wide present divergences of opinion and treatment techniques, I am convinced that such friendly interchanges would also prove mutually beneficial.

Today they are lone voices. Many would dismiss them contemptuously as the lone voices of deluded cranks yet, as I hope to show in the next chapter, they are not entirely alone, for even in the United States, England and Ireland, a tiny handful of similarly courageous trail-blazers have already produced significant testaments which it might be unwise to continue to ignore.

14. Obsession: Fact or Fantasy?

While Brazil's spirit hospitals are a new breakthrough in the world of Western medicine, it is pertinent to note that at the beginning of this century two of the keenest minds in the history of American psychic research—William James, Professor of Psychology at Harvard University (he became President of the American Society for Psychical Research in 1894–5) and James Hervey Hyslop, Professor of Logic and Ethics at Columbia University for thirteen years—had both become convinced of the reality of "obsession" as a factor to be reckoned with in mental illness.

Shortly before his death in 1910, Professor William James caustically wrote :

The refusal of modern enlightenment to treat obsession as a hypothesis to be spoken of as even possible, in spite of the massive human tradition based on concrete experience in its favour, has always seemed to me a curious example of the power of fashion in things "scientific". That the demon theory (not necessarily a devil theory) will have its innings again is to my mind absolutely certain. One has to be "scientific" indeed to be blind and ignorant enough not to suspect any such possibility.

Professor Hyslop was also fascinated by the mysteries of the psyche, particularly the seemingly linked phenomena of multiple personality and obsession.

Like his famous fellow-researcher, William James, Hyslop

conducted many experiments and carried out much research before he, too, finally and most reluctantly ceded intellectual acceptance.

In *Life after Death* he wrote:

Before accepting such a doctrine, I fought against it for ten years after I was convinced that survival after death was proved. But several cases forced upon me the consideration of the question. The chief interest in such cases is their revolutionary effect in the field of medicine. . . . It is high time for the medical world to wake up and learn something.

Nandor Fodor* tells us that the case which finally convinced Professor Hyslop concerned a distracted Brooklyn goldsmith, a Mr F. L. Thompson, who had sought Hyslop's help when he feared he was going mad. Thompson's troubles had begun six months after the death of Robert Swain Gifford, a well-known American artist. Apart from a slight interest in sketching in his youth, Thompson possessed no artistic talent and had hardly known Gifford. Yet suddenly, in 1905, he found himself seized with an irresistible impulse to sketch and paint in the style of the dead artist. Worse, he began to have hallucinations that he was Gifford himself. He was also plagued by visions of scenes of the neighbourhood where the artist had lived. Eventually, when he visited a posthumous exhibition of Gifford's paintings, he heard a voice whisper: "You see what I have done. Can you take up and finish my work?" Subsequently, two doctors diagnosed Thompson as paranoiac. Hyslop, however, unimpressed by the medical verdicts, took the goldsmith to three different mediums. Each sensed the influence of the dead artist. Attempts were successfully made to reason with the artist-obsessor who was finally persuaded to desist from tormenting his unfortunate victim.

Hyslop, who edited for many years the *Journal of the American Society for Psychical Research,* declared:

There is growing evidence of the fact of obsession which lies at the basis of much insanity and can be cured. The medical world will have to wake up and give attention to this problem or material medica will lose control of the subject.

* *Encyclopedia of Psychic Science.*

In one of his last books, *Contact With the Other World,* he again refers to the subject in the following passages :

The existence of evil spirits affecting the living is as clearly taught in the New Testament, and implied in the Old Testament, as any doctrine there expounded.

... The term obsession is employed by psychic researchers to denote the abnormal influence of spirits on the living. ... The cures effected have required much time and patience, the use of psychotherapeutics of an unusual kind, and the employment of psychics to get into contact with the obsessing agents and thus to release the hold which such agents have, or to educate them to voluntary abandonment of their persecutions. ... Every single case of dissociation and paranoia to which I have applied cross-reference has yielded to the method and proved the existence of foreign agencies complicated with the symptoms of mental or physical deterioration. It is high time to prosecute experiments on a large scale in a field that promises to have as much practical value as any application of the scalpel and the microscope.

He also reminds us :

If we believe in telepathy we believe in a process which makes possible the invasion of a personality by someone at a distance. ... It is not at all likely that sane and intelligent spirits are the only ones to exert influence from a transcendental world. If they can act on the living there is no reason why others cannot do so as well. The process in either case would be the same; we should have to possess adequate proof that nature puts more restrictions upon ignorance and evil in the next life than this in order to establish the certainty that mischievous personalities do not or cannot perform nefarious deeds. The objection that such a doctrine makes the world seem evil applies equally to the situation in the present life.

When he died Hyslop left provision in his will for the setting up in New York of a "James H. Hyslop Foundation for the Treatment of Obsession". Dr Titus Bull, director of the Foundation for twenty years, later published his startling conclusions in a paper pedantically titled: "Analysis of Unusual Experiences in Healing Relative to Diseased Minds and Results of Materialism Foreshadowed".

He wrote:

An obsessing personality is not composed of the soul, mind and will of one disembodied being, but is, in reality, a composite personality made up of many beings. The pivot obsessor, or the one who first impinges upon the sensorium of the mortal, is generally one with little resistance to the others. He or she, therefore, becomes an easy prey to those who desire to approach a mortal in this way.

According to Dr Bull, obsessors utilize three major points of impingement on the bodies they seek to tenant: the base of the brain, the solar plexus region and the reproductive organs.

But the best-known contribution in this field, at least in the Western hemisphere, is undoubtedly Dr Carl A. Wickland's *Thirty Years Among the Dead*, published in Los Angeles in 1924.

Dr Wickland was a member of the Chicago Medical Society, the American Association for the Advancement of Science and also the National Geographic Society. The eyebrow-raising title of his book is matched by its contents which comprise documented case histories encountered in the course of thirty years' experience in the field of mental illness during which he, and his wife—the latter a gifted medium—devoted themselves to helping obsessional cases. For this purpose they founded a Psychopathic Institute in Chicago. Their husband-wife partnership must surely be one of the strangest in medical annals.

When Mrs Wickland went into trance her "controls" influenced the patients' obsessors to communicate through her body. The transfer was frequently induced, or assisted, by the method of passing a low voltage current through the body of the afflicted patient. This charge of static electricity, states Dr Wickland, did not cause discomfort to the patient, but it apparently aroused intense fear in the discarnate "lodger". Dr Wickland would then proceed to parley with the ejected "obsessor", frequently succeeding in convincing the intruder that he or she was not only injuring the particular living victim but was also actually retarding their own spiritual progress in thus posthumously seeking to strengthen their ties on earth.

Wickland describes his method of "persuasion" as follows:

Those intelligences whose reasoning faculties are alert can generally be made to realize that their situation is unusual when attention is called to the dissimilarity between their own former bodily features, hands and feet, as well as clothes, and those of the psychic—especially when the spirit is a man. Some cannot be convinced and prove so obdurate that they must be forced to leave and are taken in charge by the invisible co-workers. The transference of the mental aberration or psychosis from a patient to the psychic intermediary, Mrs Wickland, is facilitated by the use of static electricity, which is applied to the patient, frequently in the presence of the psychic. Although this electricity is harmless to the patient it is exceedingly effective, for the obsessing spirit cannot long resist such electrical treatment and is dislodged.

The major part of Dr Wickland's book is a straightforward, meticulously compiled documentary consisting of scores of case histories based on actual stenographic transcriptions of Dr Wickland's extraordinary conversations with "obsessors" during treatment sessions. They are cases selected for their interest from hundreds of similar case records filed at the Wicklands' Institute.

In his explanatory preface he bluntly states:

Spirit obsession is a fact—a perversion of a natural law and is amply demonstrable. This has been proven hundreds of times by causing the supposed insanity or aberration to be temporarily transferred from the victim to a psychic sensitive who is trained for the purpose, and by this method ascertain the cause of the psychosis to be an ignorant or mischievous spirit, whose identity may frequently be identified.

By this method and without detriment to the psychic, it has

also proved possible to relieve the victim, as well as release the entity from its condition of spiritual darkness through an explanation of the laws governing the spirit world, which the experiences to follow will demonstrate. . . .

The serious problem of alienation and mental derangement attending ignorant psychic experiments was first brought to my attention by the cases of several persons whose seemingly harmless experiences with automatic writing and the ouija board resulted in such wild insanity that commitment to asylums was necessitated. . . . Many supposedly innocent ouija board cases came to my notice and my observations led me into research in psychic phenomena for a possible explanation of these strange occurrences. The influence of these discarnate entities is the cause of many of the inexplicable and obscure events of earth life and of a large part of the world's misery. Purity of life and motive, or high intellectuality, do not necessarily offer protection from obsession; recognition and knowledge of these problems are the only safeguards.

The physical conditions permitting this impingement are varied; such encroachment is often due to a natural and predisposed susceptibility, a depleted nervous system, or sudden shock. Physical derangements are conducive to obsession, for when the vital forces are lowered, less resistance is offered and intruding spirits are allowed easy access, although often neither mortal nor spirit is conscious of the presence of the other.

His conclusion is that many cases of so-called insanity—ranging from varying types of dementia and hysteria to kleptomania, religious and suicidal mania and even certain forms of criminality —can be traced to the influence or invasion of obsessors. Humanity, he tells us, "is surrounded by the thought influence of millions of discarnate beings who have not yet arrived at a full realization of life's higher purposes."

And in support of his heterodox contentions he prints the views of distinguished medical colleagues and fellow psychic researchers of his day.

They include a statement by Dr E. N. Webster, a specialist in mental illness, who appears to have had clairvoyant and clair-audient gifts :

I often see the spirits who cause insanity. At times I even hear their voices. Insane persons who are spoken of as hopelessly insane are frequently lost under the overwhelming control of a spirit or crowd of spirits. We frequently find by post-mortem examination that no physical disorder exists in the brain or nervous system of such persons.

Dr Webster's findings on post-mortem examinations carried out on the insane were also corroborated by Dr W. M. L. Coplin, a former director of the Bureau of Health and Charities, Philadelphia, Pennsylvania, who said:

Insanity, in most cases, is unaccompanied by any perceptible change in the brain structure. The brain of the patient, when examined under a microscope, shows absolutely nothing which differs in any way from the appearance of the brain of the perfectly sane person. . . . Something causes insanity but what it is, we do not yet know.

Dr Wickland also reminds us that even such a noted, sceptical researcher as Dr Hereward Carrington, in his book *Modern Psychical Phenomena*, had written:

It is evident . . . that spiritual "obsession" is at least a possibility which modern science can no longer disregard, while there are many striking facts in its support. This being so, its study becomes imperative—not only from the academic viewpoint but also because of the fact that hundreds and perhaps thousands of individuals are at the present moment suffering in this manner, and their relief demands some immediate investigation and cure. Once grant the theoretical possibility of actual obsession, and a whole vast field of research and investigation is opened up before us which demands all the care, skill and patience which modern enlightenment and psychological understanding can furnish.

In Dr Wickland's view, based on a considerable compilation of almost tediously repetitive evidence, the "obsessors" of modern times are confused earthbound entities who in former times were mistakenly described as "devils". Many, he tells us, are in a state of confusion; others, impelled by selfish motives, seek an earthly outlet for their unslaked desires.

Lacking physical bodies through which to carry out these earthly propensities, many discarnate intelligences are attracted to the magnetic light which emanates from mortals, and, consciously or unconsciously, attach themselves to these magnetic auras, finding an avenue of expression through influencing, obsessing or possessing human beings. Such obtruding spirits influence susceptible sensitives with their thoughts, impart their own emotions to them, weaken their will power and often control their actions, producing great distress, mental confusion and suffering.

His references to the "magnetic aura", an apparent force field of an as yet uncharted energy which surrounds human beings, has since received ample confirmation from at least two unexpected but reputable sources.

A year after Dr Wickland had published his "classic", an English doctor, Dr Walter J. Kilner (1847–1920), a member of the medical team at St Thomas's Hospital, London, published *The Human Atmosphere*, a dissertation on the human aura, copiously illustrated with drawings made from patients who had passed through his hands over a period of years.

His documented breakthrough, based on years of experimentation with hospital patients, attested that a force field exists around the human body which, though normally invisible, can under certain laboratory conditions be seen, charted and analysed. He predicted that at some future time this field would be photographed and this has been achieved by Soviet experimenters. He also declared—and his view is now shared by Soviet medical and psychic researchers—that it would provide enormous scope for more accurate medical diagnosis of all types of illness and mental disturbance.

In England there has been no sustained medical study in this field comparable to that done in Brazil's spirit hospitals or to the 30-years' teamwork of Dr Wickland and his wife.

Nevertheless, even in England, during the past half-century you can find a handful of pioneers who, in their varying ways—working in "Rescue Circles", in study groups, or in teams of healers attached to Spiritualist organizations—have carried out work which impinges directly, or indirectly, upon "obsessor" theories.

In the 1930s, a group of four London doctors decided to try out Dr Wickland's methods on selected patients. These experiments were described by Dr Oscar Parkes, a member of the medical quartet, in a lecture he gave in May, 1935 to London Spiritualists. The lecture was subsequently summarized in an article published in *Light* (May 23, 1935) under the title: "Doctors and Obsession Cures Effected in London on Basis of Spirit Theory".

It told how, in two cases described by Dr Parkes, the procedure followed by Dr Wickland of passing "strong charges of static electricity" into the body of the patient had produced successful results: in one instance after the medium had been thrown into violent physical convulsions and in the other without physical disturbance.

Dr Parkes also commented that much of the symptomatology of war neuroses suggested "obsession or possession by spirits of dead soldiers unconscious of their transition".

He added that the spirit hypothesis regarding war neuroses was further evidenced by the rapid recovery of patients under severe electric treatment, as instituted by Dr Vincent, who had demonstrated that it could cure in a few hours cases which had baffled psychiatrists for months.

While he himself did not believe "obsession" was a "common cause of lunacy", he stated that when all allowances had been made for those types of insanity which might be due to disease, damage, shock, etcetera, he thought there still remained a residue of cases "for which we cannot find a possible or probable cause unless we care to account for them on the lines of the effects of reincarnation or the action of the subconscious mind, especially in those cases we call border-line."

He then outlined his joint experiences with three doctor colleagues, of the use of a high tension static electric charge from a Wilmhurst machine to drive out "obsessing" entities. He said he could not explain why such electric shocks should be unbearable for the obsessing entity, but quoted the following account, as given to Dr Wickland by a spirit entity who had been dislodged from the body of a patient and who had afterwards communicated his experience through Mrs Wickland's mediumship:

I have been so strange for a long time. What in the world is it? It has been so strange at times. There was lightning and thunder, and it bothered me terribly. I have not been left alone for one minute. It was fierce that thunder and lightning. The lightning was the worst—the thunder was not so bad. The lightning is so bad that it doesn't seem as if I should really see afterwards. I should say it was coming down in torrents. It seemed as if you had got knocked on the head and then got it again and again. It was wonderful how you got it. It was a wonder, for it woke me up. It woke me up good and plenty at times, so that I could stand it no longer.

Expressing the hope that in view of the successful results he and his colleagues were obtaining, this might induce the medical profession to reconsider their adamant rejection of the spirit theory, he explained what he meant by the terms "possession" and "obsession".

By possession I mean the condition of a patient whose mind is under the control of an influence or influences which are not of this world. Obsession may be described as partial possession —there is not control to the extent of the entity of the patient being submerged into that of the possessing influence, but only that certain phases of his mentality may be influenced.

Replying to critics who claimed that "suggestion" must have played a major role in the treatment outlined, Dr Parkes countered this view by remarking that this obvious therapeutical method had failed in all the cases treated by his group. He stressed that these cases had been regarded by doctors as incurable, yet by using Dr Wickland's method they had been able to restore patients "to complete sanity. That, after all, was the supreme test!"

SERIAL CONSCIOUSNESS

It should be noted that Dr Parkes, although personally convinced of the *reality* of the psychic phenomenon of "obsessors", did not share the view held by Dr Wickland and other researchers I have earlier quoted, that it is necessarily a *common* cause of lunacy.

Similarly, another noted present-day English quester, Edwin Butler, a former Congregational minister, with nearly 25 years' practical experience of "rescue work", also has reservations of a rather different kind which are also worthy of close consideration and further testing.

Mr Butler's practical work in healing and "rescue" circles— carried out in latter years with the co-operation of his wife, a talented, courageous, trance medium—has led him to formulate a sophisticated refinement of currently accepted reincarnation theories. Outlining his views in three notable articles published in *Psychic News* during July, 1960 Mr Butler explains how he came to abandon the term "reincarnation", which he regards as a misnomer, and to coin the substitute "Serial Consciousnesss", which he regards as a more nearly true description of our fate as survivors in other worlds.

His reincarnation "heresy" was sparked off many years ago when the spirit control of a male trance medium had informed him that the troubles of a difficult patient were rooted in a former life. The communicator emphasized, however, that the spirit entity which had been brought through the medium in this particular instance was *not* an "obsessing" or "alien" personality to be "cast out", but was a "previous consciousness" of the patient which required to be reintegrated or "persuaded into harmony with the present personality".

I am not competent to interpret for the reader the full complexities of Mr Butler's thought-provoking theory. If I understand him aright, however, he likens human *personality* to the segment of an orange, in that it is essentially only a section or facet of a larger "whole", which he terms "*the individual*".

As a *personality* on this earth, each human being is unique and Mr Butler believes we continue the spiritual evolution of that *personality* in the spirit world after earthly death. We do not, he says, reincarnate back to earth under any new "personality" alias, neither apparently can we justifiably claim former "personality" incarnations in the guise of any "Cleopatras" or "Napoleons", though our evolutionary destiny will increasingly interact *with* and *upon* other *related* "personalities" in our respective *individualities*. And we will enjoy specially close Karmic links with the succeeding "segment" or "new personality" projected by our "individual" group whole, or *"higher self"*.

The importance of Mr Butler's theory in the present context of consideration of healing therapeutics in relation to apparent cases of "obsession" is the problem it raises of ascertaining whether the disorder arises from an "alien" obsessor who needs to be expelled, or an "over-intrusive previous consciousness" which is *not* alien and therefore needs to be integrated, not expelled.

For this reason Mr Butler has serious and understandable reservations about electric shock therapy—whether it takes the form of Dr Wickland's use of static electricity or the E.C.T. (electro-convulsive-therapy) used with frequent success by the medical profession. He tells me : "Electrical treatment can be used to expel an alien intruder. I do not favour its use for this purpose, though I admit it works."

Describing it as a "blunderbuss technique", he comments : "I would not myself employ it, for three reasons :

1. I do not know enough about possible side-effects on the patient. Even careful control by medical experts in the field would not satisfy me that no harm could possibly result upon at least two of the patient's 'other vehicles'—the etheric body and the aura. I have no evidence that harm *does* result, especially with a doctor who is quite sure about *exactly* what the diagnosis is, and *exactly* what shock will do, but I, personally, would not assume the risk that harm might result, in my hands.

2. Though the electricity *expels* the intruder, it does not *control* the expelled intruder : in Dr Carl Wickland's cases, the expelled intruders were under the control (apparently) of his spirit co-operators. My contention is that if the co-operating spirits are competent to control the expelled intruder, then they ought to be able to expel him in the first instance and this, for me, would be the only satisfactory evidence that I could rely on their competence.

3. There is no way in which I can distinguish between an intruding *alien* entity and an over-intrusive 'previous consciousness' (which is *not* alien and therefore must be integrated and not expelled) except by the diagnosis of my spirit helpers.

The reasons for the success of electro-convulsive-therapy by the medical profession are, in my opinion, variants of the following possibilities :

(a) a lucky bang;

(b) an accurate application of electrical interference to counteract disordered electrical activity of the brain;

(e) the expulsion of an alien intruder, not usually by intention.

Doctors are becoming increasingly reliable with (b) and maintaining their 'chance averages' with (a) and (c)."

15. A "Wonder-Working" Scientist Priest

"I suppose that I have already attended about 20,000 patients, but I am not a saint, nor do I perform miracles. I merely count upon Divine help for the cures I have been able to effect."

This characteristic disclaimer comes from a remarkable Brazilian priest, Padre Ponciano Stenzel Dos Santos, of the Parish of Our Lady of Mercy in Piedade, one of Rio de Janeiro's poorer suburbs.

A former Catholic Deputy in Brazil's parliament, this scholar-orator, a man in his late sixties, has a warrior's profile, eyes which can flash and sparkle as eloquently as his tongue and a boisterous schoolboy laugh. He is said to have turned down the offer of an archbishopric, preferring to devote his days and many of his nights to treating the sick, the mentally afflicted and the tormented.

Founder of a controversial "Institute for Psychological Research and Assistance", Padre Ponciano may be said literally to live on the job for he has transformed the major part of his shabbily elegant eighteenth-century presbytery into a treatment clinic unique in the Roman Catholic domain.

Ponciano's home crests a cobbled slope, the Rua da Capela, which has now been nicknamed the "Hill of Faith" because daily pilgrimages of patients converge upon his house at all hours of the day and night. Crowding the benches which line the sun-dappled, tree-shaded, marbled terrace, they chat cheerfully as they wait their turn for treatment, confident that none will ever be rejected on grounds of class, creed, colour, crime or lack of cash.

The Padre's highly unorthodox therapeutic treatments have frequently achieved headlines in the Brazilian press in which they have been described in terms ranging from "witchcraft" and "electronic wonder-working" to "fantastic" and "miraculous".

He became a renewed focus of controversy in the spring of 1965 when police officials invaded his home and clinic, following a complaint laid by a Brazilian doctor that Ponciano was practising "illegal medicine". An Army doctor-colonel who happened to be present during the raid, protested vigorously. He told the police he had himself been cured of a paralytic condition and offered to testify on his friend's behalf in court under oath.

Ponciano remained unperturbed. Plentifully endowed with the rebellious courage characteristic of those born in Brazil's southernmost "cowboy" state of Rio Grande do Sul, the gaucho priest has survived several appearances before frowning medical and theological commissions. He continues to insist : "I do not trespass upon the cornfields of others. My house is open to all who seek my help or wish to make any investigation. I challenge those who accuse me to debate round a table the results of my work."

Content to be described as a scientist-priest, Ponciano, a modest man, is reluctant in private conversation to talk about the healing "successes" which have brought him unsought fame. They are said to include the healing of epileptics, paralytics, heart disease, neuroses, obsession, deafness and other medically resistant ills.

Regarding himself merely as a channel for healing through "divine grace" he has told reporters that his so-called "miraculous" cures merely confirm the affirmation of Saint Paul who wrote in his First Epistle to the Corinthians :

... the manifestation of the Spirit is given to each individual for the common good, because to one the same spirit imparts the expression of wisdom ... by the same spirit another is given the gift of healing.

Readily and fully accepting that the Spirit "bloweth where it listeth", the Padre jolted many of his more orthodox-minded viewers when, on a television programme, he fearlessly defended José Arigó, fellow Roman Catholic twice imprisoned for carrying out his mission of psychic surgery.

When he was later questioned by Getulio Barro, a Brazilian journalist*, Ponciano explained :

* *Manchete* (27. 11. 65.)

Many were surprised by what I said about him ... but it is indisputable that this man does extraordinary things. He performs cures and does good without any thought of personal gain. After all, we know that there exist special powers, given by God to certain people, directly or through an intermediary angel or spirit. It is with such powers that they perform cures. What we cannot do is to lift ourselves against God. If there are doubts, then carry out an investigation. The laws of science can be applied to everything. And beyond science lies the Divine Power, a breath of the Holy Spirit.

Tolerant in outlook and quick to applaud dedication and courage in another human being, Padre Ponciano also stressed:

José Arigó performs his cures with use of a kitchen knife, some cotton-wool and calling on God's blessing. I rehabilitate my patients by means of an electronic chair, also calling upon Divine Grace. ... As in the case of Arigó, I am also at peace. One has nothing to fear when we live for others.

Defining psycho-electronics as representing the links between our consciousness and electro-magnetic currents, Padre Ponciano speaks with an authority which rests upon decades of study.

He says: "For some thirty years I have dedicated myself to psychology and I have reached the conclusion that the natural and supernatural worlds are not separated. For this reason materialistic psychology cannot solve man's problems. On the other hand, I have also observed that illnesses, particularly nervous illnesses, do not stem from microbes or bacteria, but from the loss of electrons. When we lose electrons the chemistry of the body is altered. If there is an increase of electrons, the chemistry also alters, but in a positive or beneficial manner."

Ponciano remains an addictive patient researcher. When I had the pleasure of visiting him on several occasions in January, 1967, he brought out from his well-stocked library an impressive selection of books relating to his current delvings in the fields of mind exploration and parapsychological research. They included: Harvey Elliott White's *Introduction to Atomic Spectra*; Pierre

Daco's *Les Prodigies et Les Victoires De La Psychologie*; Alfred Still's *On the Frontiers of Science and Parapsychology*; a Portuguese translation of Dr Rhine's *New Frontiers of the Mind*, and *Truth is Indivisible* by J. Herculiano Pires, a distinguished Brazilian lawyer-medium. Although the Padre affirms with the trace of a twinkle that his scientific work comes well within the permitted orbit of the scholastic psychology of St Thomas of Aquinas, he is a sterner critic of modern seers. He certainly praises Freud for having done so much valuable pioneer work in dispelling the medieval theological dictum that the victims of psychic disorders were possessed by the devil or paying for frightful sins, and for having with his genius paved the way to important conquests in the field of mind exploration. But as a philosopher he dismisses Freud as mediocre. "He denied spiritual forces," says the healer priest, "and here Freud erred. It is not possible to deny what is spiritual".

A true citizen of the world, the priest's scientific studies led him first to France and later to India and Japan. Journalists have written much about Ponciano's use in healing of a so-called "electronic" chair, developed by a Japanese doctor and a Japanese engineer, both of Tokyo University. Invented and constructed by Dr T. Fujiyama and Dr T. Ouchi, the priest's "magnetizer" chair is an ingenious apparatus which, it is claimed, effectively utilizes the curative properties of ultra-long waves. Ponciano first saw this type of apparatus at Hiroshima.

He tells us that when the current is switched on magnetism is produced by a resulting transformation of electric fields. He says this process enables: "Long waves of 6,000 metres to penetrate into the bone even more effectively than do X-rays. At the same time there is a bodily restoration of the electrons which are lost with earth contact through the feet, either from fatigue or other disorders which I am still studying."

One of the first volunteers to test the chair at the priest's clinic was Franciso José de Carvalho, a journalist from the state of Amazonas. Carvalho was suffering from a nervous breakdown after spending eight months in the Equatorial jungle. When doctors in Manaus failed to ameliorate his suffering he decided to place himself under the priest's care. Two months later he was able to resume active life. Another striking case reported was that of Benedito Ramos Junior, a paralytic from Angra dos Reis who had to be carried into the priest's home. A fortnight later he demonstrated his improvement by running the entire circumference of the padre's church.

But Padre Ponciano, a man of profound insights, does not content himself solely with the discoveries of science, whether these be expressed within the covers of learned textbooks or in the outward form of technical apparatus.

While he believes that man's nervous system and even his physical heart comprise "spirally interlinked electro-magnetic circuits", he also holds the view that : "In this world we might also be in contact with other worlds of different frequencies."

Certainly his own intensive study of the paranormal, particularly the complex psychological and psychic riddles of mediumship displayed daily in manifold forms throughout the length and breadth of his homeland, has imbued him with a profound respect for the mysterious and frequently regenerative powers of the incarnate mind as expressed in hynotically-induced deep trance states.

He himself makes therapeutic use of hypnosis. He has publicly stated : "Through hypnotic sleep I suggest to the patient that he should bury all negative memories and I instil into his subconscious positive impulses." Ponciano never administers orthodox medical drugs of any kind, preferring his own frequently very effective combination of prayer and hypnotic therapy.

And he makes no secret of the fact that he unhesitatingly utilizes the psychic powers of a woman trance medium as a diagnostic aid in his preliminary analysis of psychological and nervous disorders. Her help enables him to complete what might be termed an instant psychoanalysis of a patient within the incredibly short space of time of seven or eight minutes. He told me: "I use Mme. M.'s clairvoyance rather like a TV aerial to get relevant images and information."

Certainly it was fascinating to watch the speed with which the entranced medium, a pleasant, middle-aged housewife with no medical knowledge, was able to reel off answers to a list of questions asked by the priest as he held a printed chart upon which he recorded her varied observations on the patient in code form. I noted that the questions included inquiries relating to the influence of "stars", "planets", "spirit entities", parental conditions and material problems. The priest had earlier induced instantaneous deep trance in Mme M. by means of a previously implanted post-hypnotic suggestion which took the visible form of gently nipping the lobe of her left ear as she sat relaxed, her bare feet touching the floor, in a chair next to the patient being treated.

Mme M.'s trance capacities also apparently include out-of-body-travel which some researchers term "distant clairvoyance". The padre told me how on one occasion he had wished to alleviate a German patient's deep anxiety about his wife's health. "I gave Mme M. the address of the man's home in Hamburg and to test whether she was really there out-of-body, I asked her to describe the house to me. She gave details of a two-storied dwelling and a basement which were accepted as correct by my patient. Then she went on to tell us 'I see a fat lady'. My patient intervened at this point and said, 'That's wrong. My wife is thin.' When I asked Mme M. to explain this error of trance imagination she tranquilly continued : 'This lady who is fat is not the wife but a line leads from her to a hospital where the fat lady visits his wife.' I asked her to 'follow the line' and to describe the wife's condition. She then told us : 'Her illness is not serious. When he returns she will get well.' " The business-man, who had been planning to extend his trip by another four months, returned home immediately. He later wrote to tell Ponciano that his wife had quickly recovered, as predicted. He also confirmed that at the time of the Rio experiment a plump woman friend had indeed been staying in his home and visiting the hospital where his wife had been a patient.

16. Pedro the Bridge-Builder

Memorable encounters with Pedro McGregor, a deceptively mild-mannered Cariocan, born in Rio de Janeiro on Christmas Eve, 1931, remind me of Brazil's favourite firewater tipple, Cachaça. This deadly distillation of the sugar cane—its very name glissades invitingly over the tongue as casha-a-s-a—is visually the innocuous twin of tap water, but crescendos down the increasingly aghast gullet like a Vesuvius in liquid eruption.

And so it is as you listen with deepening attention to this dynamic young-old, journalist-psychic researcher, or watch him in action as the unpaid "pastor" of a healing centre, sited not far away from the sun-diamonded beaches which are favourite playgrounds for millionaires as well as paupers.

A meeting with him in Rio became a "must" for me after I had read with ever deepening interest his stimulating book, cryptically titled *The Moon and Two Mountains*. Launched simultaneously in London and Toronto in 1966, and later in the United States, a sub-title describes the contents as : *The Myths, Ritual and Magic of Brazilian Spiritism*. Textually this is strictly true, even if a trifle off-putting, like the author's own eloquent lapses into frowning silence whenever conversation veers too closely towards the personal. But it is the metaphysical conclusions he draws from his 15 years' questing which pack a punch for complacent orthodox thinking, whether this relates to racial problems, philosophy, science or religion.

At the time of our first meeting in December, 1967, Pedro, companioned by Astor, his devoted Alsatian dog, was living in a simply furnished eighth-floor apartment in Ipamena, an attractive beach suburb of Brazil's capital. Book-lined shelves of meticulously indexed books bore eloquent witness to unorthodox quests little favoured by the conventionally ambitious, money-greedy or power-lusting. Here within the well-thumbed covers, were the varied fuels which had stoked the voracious intellectual appetite of their owner, a man blessed with a computer-memory.

Proud of his Scottish ancestry, his music-loving, intellectual parents and his native country Brazil, Pedro was educated in a Jesuit seminary where, at the age of 14, he revelled in Plato's *Dialogues on Immortality,* Dante's *Inferno* and the wisdom of Aristotle. Gifted with a precocious intelligence, he became tormented by philosophical doubts which found no easy answers when he later came to Europe to attend courses at King's College, Cambridge, the London School of Economics and others in Vienna. When he returned home he first tried banking as a career but didn't like it. Eventually he found a more congenial niche as a political columnist for Brazilian national newspapers, and later as an international correspondent and researcher for European and American journals.

Twice married—his first marriage ended in divorce, the second in death—he became increasingly engrossed in researches devolving on the philosophic, scientific and occult mysteries of Brazil's aboundingly rich theogonic mosaic expressed in the "twin mountains" of Spiritist and Umbandist movements, each claiming millions of devotees.

His resulting book, which I venture to predict will become an increasingly valued source of reference for generations of psychical researchers, admirably portrays that it is no chance happening that in Brazil today we may well be witnessing the birth of a psychically-gifted nation and culture, sired by miscegenation, and mothered amid centuries of slavery, colonization and suffering. In the words of Pedro McGregor:

The Portuguese and the African Negro came from afar to meet in Brazil and together with the Indian form there a new people, a new civilization with a different personality. In a unique way, different ancestries and levels of culture found in Brazil the catalyst which formed them into an amalgam that carries within itself the fundamental elements of spiritual greatness: the Brazilian people.

No other people has such deeply inbred religious feeling completely above all doctrine and dogma; no other people has such simple, sincere and friendly feelings towards its fellow men, whatever their race, creed or colour, and no other people whose culture is of Western extraction has such a flair for magic and the supernatural.

Several factors contributed to this. The colonists were initiated in magic practice by the Moors, the Mediterranean African Negroes and the European alchemists, while remaining themselves at the same time stoutly Catholic. This paradoxical combination of influences was enriched further in the colony, where the influence of the Church was diluted by distance and the eclecticism of the cultural scene increased by miscegenation, first with Indian, then with African women. The humility and simplicity of the Negro in his religious devotion was passed on to the Portuguese through African nurses and mistresses, the resulting blend being a mixture of Catholicism and fetichism. . . .

Throughout his years of research McGregor has observed a golden rule. He told me : "In psychical research you have to be careful to keep both the phenomenon studied and your reasoning about it parallel so that you can separate what is actually dynamic law and some higher force in action, and what is individualized in the people practising the phenomenon. You must also have the keen eye and objectivity of the reporter-sociologist in which you don't take anything for granted. It is like a painful laboratory research when you have to deal with many fundamental, seemingly unrelated events which you slowly try to piece together, groping always towards a sensed but unperceived pattern. And you must never be dogmatic."

He described his own personal progress to his present viewpoint and developed mediumship as a slow and painful process of trial and error. "I experienced no mystic blaze of illumination. Neither did I find the answers I sought in conventional ways of living, working, marrying, and spending. I knocked my head against many obstacles and slowly learned the hard way how things tick. I also learned not to blame the world but to seek what was wrong in myself. In this way I didn't develop grudges, but continued groping, exploring, suffering, until one day I found the picture whole !"

Where McGregor made his leap of genius as a sociological

psychic researcher was in his realization that what was still lacking in Brazil was an umbrella, a framework within which, as he rightly says, conflicting, yet linked practices, could be accommodated. "If the divine is indeed factual, there must be an explanation embracing all of them, in all their aspects, and rejecting none, which yet accords with the laws of science."

He first attempted to translate his theories into practice by opening in 1958, his first Temple in fashionable Ipamena. A twenty-foot neon sign proclaimed to myriads of passing cars and beach promenaders: *Temple of Universal Religion*. A smaller sign reads: *Religion at the Service of Science*.

It was not long before long queues of people each Tuesday evening patiently awaited their turn to enter the large room where some thirty mediums, all dressed in white, sat around a long table, holding hands to establish a "current". Here, headed by Pedro, standing at the head of the table, the mediums received spiritual entities of a homely character, the "Cabocles or old negroes" formerly only welcome in Umbandist circles. The main purpose of these unusual healing sessions, he tells us, was to counter the ill-effects of black magic, the "evil eye", malign influences and "bad spiritual company".

He defines "Universal Religion" as the first attempt in Brazil to work towards a unification of the Spiritist movement, not through any kind of Pope or any kind of imposed structure, "but simply by harmonizing the various currents of thought and of spiritual principle in conformity with the laws of nature and not with preconceived ideas or ancient religious traditions, however valuable."

For McGregor, dogmas and "miracles" are out. He believes that material energy is basically a condensation of spiritual energy. He himself claims to have witnessed remarkable physical phenomena in his psychic researches. He described one instance when the radiance emanating from a materialized form was so great it had illuminated the seance room. "I felt as if I wanted to throw myself down before it." Psychic power, he says, is a universal, neutral energy, which can be used for good or ill though the man who seeks to misuse it will be asking for trouble, in the same way that an alcoholic who drives a car becomes accident-prone. In his view no training can enhance the degree of psychic power possessed by an individual but it *can* enhance its quality and service to others. In a training lecture he gave one evening to his team of young mediums I heard him describe mediumship as a "true diamond" which must be polished to enable it to reflect back its full brilliance. "If we are given this diamond and are sceptical about its true worth; if we throw it in the mud; then the diamond can be mistaken for a crystal, it will continue to give out brilliance, but not with maximum clarity and purity."

Likening clairvoyance to a television set, he told them : "What the medium does is to transform electric current but the end result will depend upon the quality of the machine. If the instrument has faulty valves it is obvious it will produce a distorted image. Now the cost of a television engineer is quite expensive when a set breaks down. It is also very expensive for a medium to rectify an image which has come out wrong through his fault. So a medium must seek to perfect his own instrument 'himself' so that the image he transmits can be as clear and as true as possible."

Later I was privileged to attend one of the twice weekly healing sessions held in Pedro's healing temple which continued to attract hundreds of patients. The session I attended was devoted to cleansing or discharging "negative" currents from the auric field around the physical body.

For centuries, the existence of such a field has been proclaimed by mediums, mystics and even by artists in religious paintings when they have depicted symbolic haloes around the heads of saints and angels. Clairvoyants and spiritual healers have also stressed that the psychically-seen auric field around the living body accurately reflects prevailing emotional, character and health conditions.

The first Western doctor who wrote a scientific study of the auric field surrounding human beings was an Englishman, Dr Walter J. Kilner of St Thomas's Hospital, London, who published the result of his researches in a book which deserves to be much more widely known. Titled *The Human Atmosphere* it was first published in 1911, followed by a revised, enlarged edition in 1920. Kilner was also an investigator in the electrical field. He tells us :

The discovery of a screen making the aura visible was by no means accidental. After reading about the action of the rays upon phosphorescent sulphide of calcium, the writer was for a long time experimenting upon mechanical forces of certain bodily emanations and had come to the conclusion, whether rightly or wrongly, that he had detected two forces beside heat that could act upon his needles, and that these forces were situated in the infra-red portion of the spectrum.

In the early part of 1908 he hit upon Dicyanin, a coal tar dye, as a substance which might make some portion of the above effects visible, in which case he expected to see the human aura. Kilner succeeded beyond his wildest dreams. In his documented record of hundreds of subsequent experiments, copiously illustrated with diagrams of the aura, he demonstrated that no two persons have identical auras. He also revealed that the human aura comprised three distinct parts.

First there is a transparent dark space, not exceeding quarter of an inch, surrounding and adjacent to the body. This he called "the etheric double". Then there is an inner aura: "It is the densest portion and varies comparatively little, or even not at all in width, either at the back, front, or sides, and in both males and females."

The third portion, or outer aura, he described as inconstant in size. Kilner also established that changes occur in the aura's size and shape. He was firmly convinced that scientific study of the aura would enhance accuracy in medical diagnosis. It is also important to note that while he declined to be dogmatic in his theories, he frankly described the series of experiments which had led him to renounce an earlier belief that the auric force was either electro-magnetic in origin, or due to radio-activity as then known.

Now Kilner's work has been confirmed from a surprising quarter. In the early 1960s Soviet developments in "lightless" microphotography produced sensational photographs which provide further scientific proof of the human aura. In the summer of 1962, a two-page article, published in a Moscow magazine *Soviet Union*, was illustrated with astonishing colour photographs of "flares of life" emanating from various sections of the human body, including the chest and fingers. They also included a series showing progressively fading "flares of life" in a dying plant. I. Leonidov, writer of the article, revealed that research establishments had been created to study the phenomenon. He commented that Soviet experts believed: "The new method will make it possible to investigate many secrets of life; it will make it possible to diagnose diseases much earlier than at present." This prediction, if proved true, will fulfil the dream of Dr Kilner who had written half a century earlier:

"I am certain that a photographic picture of the size, shape and condition of the human aura is not only possible but will shortly be made, thus enabling the aura to become a still greater assistance in medical diagnosis. It has been my earnest desire to achieve this object but now, age with its attendant infirmities, superadded to other difficulties, almost precludes any hope."

Clairvoyant auric diagnosis, of course, has long been an important factor in Western spiritual healing. Auric "cleansing" or toning up by means of healing passes administered by a medium is also widely used in many forms of spiritual healing, not only in Brazil, both in Spiritist and Umbandist healing sessions, but also in Europe and North America.

In *The Moon and Two Mountains*, McGregor tells us:

The motivating force drawing most people to spiritism in the first instance is undoubtedly therapeutic—to obtain cures denied by orthodox medicine. The principal media through which these are obtained are the so-called "fluidified water", magnetic "passes" whereby mediums wholly or partially under the control of guides remove "negative" magnetic particles from the body and replace them with "positive" particles, homoeopathic prescriptions and "invisible" operations. "Fluidified water" is that which has been submitted to the outstretched hands of the medium, through which the spirits pass into the water other fluids of a magnetic, spiritual nature specifically designed to cure the body's ills or at least alleviate them. The technique, of course, appears totally removed from any known principle or scientific nomenclature, but that is not to say that it does not work.

In his pioneering efforts to bridge the wide gulf between scientific and religious thinking Pedro McGregor has, I think, made a notable step forward. Instead of traditional healing passes made around the body of an individual patient by a medium, he has endeavoured to weld the spiritual and psychic powers of a team of mediums—they can number as many as ten or fifteen mediums acting in concert under his direction—in the form of what I can only describe as a linked human battery. The effects so obtained can be startling to watch, but the queues of patients who have attended his healing sessions over the years would appear to provide living testimony to the apparent efficacy of the method.

On the evening I was present each patient on arrival was handed a numbered disc entitling the individual to treatment when his or her number was called out.

Admitted in batches of about a dozen, well over 100 patients had been treated that evening before I had to leave around ten o'clock, and a few score still remained patiently. When my own turn came I and my companions were shown into the large treatment room where the mediums were already seated around a long table. The majority of them seemed to be already in trance. We were silently escorted to standing places behind and between the mediums and asked to grasp the upraised hands of the mediums to our left and right. Thus we created a linked chain. Classical music continued to be softly relayed from a radiogram by the door. Incense burned in open saucers placed on the table and on the windowsill of an open window.

When the human battery had been formed Pedro McGregor, who stood at the head of the table, chanted a brief invocatory prayer of thanksgiving to God. At the third repetition of the invocation he made a sweeping gesture with his hand and a great current of energy seemed to pass through the bodies and palms of the mediums into those of the patients. Where a medium appeared to be needing additional assistance Pedro silently moved towards the medium and placed his hands around the head of the patient who appeared to be the source of the trouble. He did so in my case and I was conscious of a current which appeared to flow through his hands.

After the healing he silently motioned me to sit in a chair near the table to enable me to observe subsequent "discharge" healings. One of them I am unlikely ever to forget. During the healing Pedro had gone to the help of a young medium who appeared to be in great distress. One of her hands was held by a saturnine-looking man who appeared to be in a dazed and semi-tranced condition himself. Afterwards Pedro directed the attendant to clear the room of all patients except this one man who then became the sole recipient of the entire force generated by the team of mediums who all linked hands, while Pedro additionally placed his own hands around the man's head. As the current ran through the human battery, following Pedro's triply chanted invocation, a great wave of sorrow appeared to sweep through all the mediums, expressed in an anguished groan. The young medium who had formerly evidenced distress again appeared to be the most affected and threshed her body from side to side as if seeking to break contact. No questions are ever asked of any patient during "discharge" sessions but I later learned that the patient who had been singled out for additional help was believed to be an assassin for whom the police were searching.

Through a friendly intermediary I talked to several patients at the temple, as they sat relaxed and chatting in the patio or partook of cooling drinks and light refreshments served for a modest charge from a small buffet. Others strolled in the rear garden in the warm night where candles flickered in the slight night breeze—each symbolizing an invocation for healing help, as in Roman Catholic churches.

Larry Carr, a former Hollywood actor who had also played many arduous roles in a number of Brazilian films, told me that when he had first arrived in Brazil he had been a near nervous wreck who had become completely sceptical about orthodox psychiatry when a succession of expensive practitioners had failed to find the cause and cure for his condition.

The first Rio film for which he had signed up included a scene based on an Umbandist healing centre. He became interested. A man of considerable physical courage, he had on one occasion accepted a challenge from an Umbandist medium to "walk on broken glass". He faithfully followed the medium's instructions and survived the ordeal without physical injury. He told me : "I experienced no harm or pain. I only felt pressure on the soles of my feet." He assured me : "Of course I could only do it in the presence of this medium fellow when he had given the word for me to step on the broken glass strewn over the ground. I heard of a woman who had thought she could do it alone to prove it was merely a trick. Boy, did she land up in hospital !"

At the time I became acquainted with Larry he was a handsome six-footer in superb physical and mental health. He had been healed at the temple and was now developing his own healing gifts as a useful member of Pedro's multi-racial team of mediums.

"Here in Rio," he told me, "I have at last found something

which has an element of truth. At this temple I feel at ease. There are no charges made, no questions asked, and no religious dogmas. Our work here is primarily to help people—human beings who are in a hell of a mess as I was."

17. Seer of the Psyche

Carl Gustav Jung, seer of the psyche, was a man always thoroughly at home with the unexpected and even the incredible. "The difference between most people and myself," he has told us, "is that for me the 'dividing walls' are transparent. That is my peculiarity. Others find these walls so opaque that they see nothing behind them and therefore think nothing is there. To some extent I perceive the processes going on in the background and that gives me an inner certainty."

This self-description in his autobiographical *Memories, Dreams, Reflections,* reluctantly commenced in his eighty-third year, could well serve as an apt definition of mediumship. And this is not so surprising, for in the pages of this remarkable testament it becomes amply evident that from an early age his own life contained an abundance of supernormal experiences.

Decades earlier, when Jung had attended a wedding feast, accompanied by his young wife, he had found himself involved in a discussion on criminal psychology with a middle-aged barrister who was a total stranger to him. In lively discussion, and wishing to reinforce a point on criminal psychology, Jung had made up a story around a fictional character. As he proceeded with his fancies, silence fell upon surrounding guests and a strange expression came over the face of the obviously embarrassed protagonist. Jung was puzzled and abashed, particularly when a mutual friend later chided him for his unfeeling "indiscretion". To his own horrified amazement he learned that he had unwittingly told the true story of the stranger's life. Yet Jung was never able later to recall a single word of his inadvertent verbal bombshell.

The incident made him realize afresh that he, too, abundantly possessed, like his own psychically gifted mother, what he has termed a No 2 Personality. This had enabled her at times to speak with an austere prescience which, he says, "always struck to the core of my being".

In the prologue to his autobiographical revelations Jung wrote : "My life is a story of the self-realization of the unconscious. . . . In the end the only events in my life worth telling are those when the imperishable world irrupted into this transitory one." And therein, perhaps, lies the secret of his genius as a psychiatrist or, as he himself has termed it, a doctor-of-the-soul.

Indeed, his own questing curiosity which led him to the farthest bounds of human thought, and frequently beyond the academically acceptable, may in part be traced to two striking psychic incidents in his early manhood. The first occured during the summer holidays of 1908 when he had already begun his medical studies at the University of Basle. Sitting in a room adjoining a dining room where his mother sat knitting, both were startled to hear a report like a pistol shot. A large family dining table, made of finest seasoned walnut, had suddenly split from its rim to beyond the centre. The second happened a fortnight later when he arrived home to find his mother and a maid upset by another deafening, inexplicable report, this time from the direction of the sideboard. Examination of its interior revealed that a steel bread knife had split into four pieces. Jung took them for examination by an expert cutler who told him : "There is no fault in the steel. Someone must have deliberately broken it piece by piece. Good steel can't explode."

Jung reports that his astonishment over these incidents was as great as if the Rhine had suddenly flowed backwards. Was Jung himself a potential psychical medium? The question can be asked because years later he found himself involved in a similar psychic experience which was to have historic consequences. It happened in Vienna in 1909, when Jung had asked Freud his views on precognition and parapsychology in general. Freud, not surprisingly, had come down heavily in favour of a scathing rejection. His dismissal of the subject as nonsensical produced in Jung a curious sensation. He records : "It was as if my diaphragm were made of iron and were becoming red-hot—a glowing vault. And at that moment there was such a loud report in the bookcase, which stood right next to us, that we both started up in alarm, fearing the thing was going to topple over on us. I said to Freud :

'There, that is an example of a so-called catalytic exteriorization phenomenon.'.

" 'Oh come,' he exclaimed, 'That is sheer bosh.'

" 'It is not,' I replied. 'You are mistaken, Herr Professor. And to prove my point I now predict that in a moment there will be another loud report!' Sure enough, no sooner had I said the words than the same detonation went off in the bookcase.' "

The incident made a deep impression upon both men, in Freud's case a painful one. Jung himself believed the incident aroused his friend's mistrust of him and significantly a contemptuous reference made by Freud about the occult in a subsequent conversation the following year confirmed the growing rift in their viewpoints.

Jung tells us that the remark occurred when Freud, in seeking to extract a promise from him that he would never "abandon the sexual theory", had added, "You see, we must make a dogma of it, an unshakeable bulwark." When Jung, astonished, had asked, "A bulwark—against what?" Freud replied, "Against the black tide of mud—of occultism." Sadly recalling his alarm at Freud's use of the words "bulwark" and "dogma", Jung tells us in his autobiography : "This was the thing that struck at the heart of our friendship. I knew that I would never be able to accept such an attitude. What Freud seemed to mean by 'occultism' was virtually everything that philosophy and religion, including the rising contemporary science of parapsychology, had learned about the psyche."

If the subsequent break was inevitable, and an undoubted personal tragedy for both men, it was also profoundly fructifying, for if Freud's courageous researches led to the liberation of the libido which became a precursor to our present permissive Western societies, so, too, can Jung be deemed a pioneer liberator of man's psyche in this advancing era of Mind revolution. For Jung the horizons are limitless. He has stated :*

I can only gaze with wonder and awe at the depths and heights of our psychic nature. Its non-spatial universe conceals an untold abundance of images which have accumulated over millions of years of living development and become fixed in the organism. . . . And these images are not pale shadows, but tremendously powerful psychic factors. . . . Besides this picture

* *Freud and Psychoanalysis*, Coll. Works, Vol. 4, p. 331.

I would like to place the spectacle of the starry heavens at night, for the only equivalent of the universe within is the universe without; and just as I reach this world through the medium of the body, so I reach that world through the medium of the psyche.

Over the decades, with ever increasing forcefulness, he constantly emphasized the primary importance of psychic realities, and sought to hammer home the need to "see life in the round". Describing the psyche as the most powerful fact in the human world he stated : "It is indeed the mother of all human facts, of culture and of murderous wars. All this is at first psychic and imperceptible. As long as it remains 'merely' psychic, it is not perceived by the senses, but it is nevertheless indisputably real."

In 1957, in a series of filmed interviews in Zurich with Richard I. Evans, a Texan Professor of Psychology, he also stressed, as did his nineteenth-century predecessor, Frederick Myers, that man's psychic faculties are *evolutionary*, not archaic. He told his American interviewer :

It is a fact that people develop in their psychic development on the same principle as they develop in the body. Why should we assume that it is a different principle? It is really the same kind of evolutionary behaviour as the body shows. The psyche is nothing different from the living being. It is even the psychic aspect of matter.

With far-sighted percipience he foresaw the troubles ahead for our technologically obsessed societies. He wrote :

We have plunged down a cataract of progress which sweeps us on into the future with ever wilder violence the farther it takes us from our roots. . . . We rush impetuously into novelty, driven by a mounting sense of insufficiency, dissatisfaction and restlessness. We no longer live on what we have but on promises, no longer in the light of the present day, but in the darkness of the future which, we expect, will at last bring the proper sunrise. We refuse to recognize that everything better is purchased at the price of something worse.

"Our world," said Jung, "hangs on a thin thread and that thread is the psyche of man. . . . It is not the reality of the hydrogen bomb we must fear, but what man does with it." In those haunting words he characteristically not only summated man's most exigent peril, but simultaneously pointed the way to its solution, for Jung was a man who had long recognized and lived by the truth inherent in the ancient Chinese saying: Every Wall a Door.

Bibliography

British Association/Granada Guildhall lectures, 1965, Granada Publishing and MacGibbon & Kee.

Connell, R. and Cummins, G., *Healing the Mind*, Aquarian Press, 1957.

Cummins, G., *Unseen Adventures*, Rider, 1951; *The Scripts of Cleophas*, Harold Vinal, 1928; *They Survive*, Rider, 1946; *Swan on a Black Sea*, Routledge, 1965.

Fate magazine (USA), Dr Joseph Banks Rhine, "Science and the Spiritual Nature of Man", July 1967.

Ferreira, Dr Inacio, *New Ways of Medicine; Psychiatry Face to Face with Reincarnation* (Brazil).

Fodor, Nandor, *Encyclopedia of Psychic Science*, Arthurs Press, 1933; *Between Two Worlds*, Paperback Library, 1969.

Hardy, Sir Alister, FRS, *The Living Stream*, Collins, 1966.

Hurkos, Peter, *Psychic*, Arthur Barker, 1962.

Hutton, Bernard, *Healing Hands*, W. H. Allen, 1966.

Hyslop, Prof. James Hervey, *Psychical Research and Survival*, New York, 1913; *Life After Death*, New York, 1918.

Johnson, Raynor C., *The Imprisoned Splendour*, Hodder & Stoughton, 1953; *Nurslings of Immortality*, Hodder & Stoughton, 1957; *The Light and the Gate*, Hodder & Stoughton.

Jordan, Pascual, "Parapsychological Implications of Research in Atomic Physics", *International Journal of Parapsychology*, Autumn 1960.

Journal of the Society for Psychical Research, London.

Jung, Carl Gustav, *Memories, Dreams, Reflections*, Routledge and Collins, 1963; *Freud and Psychoanalysis*, Collected Works, Vol. 4, Routledge, 1961.

Kardec, Allan, *The Spirits' Book*, Livraria Allan Kardec, São Paulo, Brazil, 1966.

Light magazine, Dr Oscar Parkes, "Doctors and Obsession Cures Effected in London on Basis of Spirit Theory", May 23, 1935.

London Hospital Gazette, March 1968.

Manchete magazine, Brazil, October 12, 1968.

McGregor, Pedro, *The Moon and Two Mountains*, Souvenir Press, 1965.

Myers, Frederic William Henry, *Human Personality and its Survival of Bodily Death*, Longmans, Green, 1903.

Psychic News, London: Serial Consciousness articles, July 1960, and Anne Dooley contributions.

Puharich, Dr Andrija, *Beyond Telepathy*, Darton, Longman & Todd, 1962.

Rhine, Dr Joseph Banks, and Pratt, J. B., *Parapsychology—Frontier Science of the Mind*, Springfield, USA, 1957.

Sargant, William, *Battle for the Mind*, Heinemann, 1957.

Sherwood, Jane, *The Psychic Bridge*, Hutchinson, 1942; *The Country Beyond*, Spearman, 1969; *The Fourfold Vision*, Spearman, 1966.

Shirokogoroff, S. M., *Psychomental Complex of the Tungus*, Kegan Paul, Trench, Trubner—Peking Edition, 1935.

Sputnik (Soviet magazine), February, 1968.

Sunday Mirror, Theo Lang articles, London, January, 1966.

Vasiliev, Prof. Leonid, *Experiments in Mental Suggestion,* Institute for the Study of Mental Images, 1967.

Wallace, Alfred Russel, *On Miracles and Modern Spiritualism*, Psychic Book Club, 1965.

Wickland, Dr Carl A., *Thirty Years Among the Dead*, Los Angeles, 1924.